Disorders of Auditory Function

Disorders of Auditory Function

Proceedings of the British Society of Audiology
First Conference—held at the University of
Dundee, from 14 to 16 July, 1971

Edited by

W. TAYLOR

Department of Social and Occupational Medicine,
University of Dundee, Scotland

PUBLISHED FOR THE BRITISH SOCIETY OF AUDIOLOGY BY

 1973

Academic Press · London · New York

ACADEMIC PRESS INC. (LONDON) LTD.
24/28 Oval Road,
London NW1

United States Edition published by
ACADEMIC PRESS INC.
111 Fifth Avenue
New York, New York 10003

Library of Congress Catalog Card Number: 72–12282
ISBN: 0–12–684750–9

PRINTED IN GREAT BRITAIN BY
COX & WYMAN LTD.
LONDON, FAKENHAM AND READING

List of Contributors

J.-M. ARAN, *Laboratoire D'Audiologie Experimentale, Faculté de Médicine de Bordeaux, Bordeaux, France.*

G. R. C. ATHERLEY, *University of Aston in Birmingham, Birmingham, England.*

B. BARR, *Department of Audiology, Karolinska, Sjukhuset, Stockholm, Sweden.*

R. M. BARR-HAMILTON, *Department of Electrical Engineering, University of Salford, Salford, England.*

H. A. BEAGLEY, *The Institute of Laryngology and Otology, London, England.*

J. BENCH, *Audiology Research Unit, Royal Berkshire Hospital, Reading, England.*

L. D. BENITEZ, *Central Institute for the Deaf, St. Louis, Missouri, U.S.A.*

V. BRASIER, *Department of Audiology and Education of the Deaf, The University, Manchester, England.*

M. E. BRYAN, *Department of Electrical Engineering, University of Salford, Salford, England.*

D. L. CHADWICK, *Department of Otolaryngology, The University, Manchester, England.*

R. R. A. COLES, *Institute of Sound and Vibration Research, University of Southampton, Southampton, England.*

M. DUNN, *School Health Service, Glasgow, Scotland.*

D. H. ELDREDGE, *Central Institute for the Deaf, St. Louis, Missouri, U.S.A.*

SIR ALEXANDER EWING, *Horseshoe Cottage, Alderley Edge, Cheshire, England.*

A. G. GIBB, *Department of Otolaryngology, University of Dundee, Dundee, Scotland.*

A. GLORIG, *The Callier Hearing and Speech Center, Dallas, Texas, U.S.A.*

G. W. GLOVER, *Department of Otolaryngology, University of Dundee, Dundee, Scotland.*

R. HINCHCLIFFE, *Institute of Laryngology and Otology, University of London, London, England.*

W. D. HINE, *Department of Audiology and Education of the Deaf, The University, Manchester, England.*

J. D. HOOD, *Institute of Neurology, The National Hospital, London, England.*

W. D. KEIDEL, *Physiologisches Institut der Universitat Erlangen-Nurnberg, Erlangen, West Germany.*

R. L. KELL, *Department of Social and Occupational Medicine, University of Wales, Cardiff, Wales. (Formerly at Department of Social and Occupational Medicine, University of Dundee, Dundee, Scotland.)*

J. J. KNIGHT, *Institute of Laryngology and Otology, University of London, London, England.*

R. K. MAL, *Ear, Nose and Throat Hospital, Glasgow, Scotland.*

A. MARKIDES, *Institute of Sound and Vibration Research, University of Southampton, Southampton, England.*

D. N. MAY, *Institute of Sound and Vibration Research, University of Southampton, Southampton, England.**

E. S. McGREGOR, *Education Department, Glasgow, Scotland.*

T. MORRIS, *Department of Audiology and Education of the Deaf, The University, Manchester, England.*

J. C. G. PEARSON, *Department of Social and Occupational Medicine, University of Dundee, Dundee, Scotland.*

C. A. POWELL, *Department of Audiology and Education of the Deaf, The University, Manchester, England.*

V. M. PRIEDE, *Institute of Sound and Vibration Research, University of Southampton, Southampton, England.*

M. PORTMANN, *Laboratoire D'Audiologie Experimentale, Faculté de Médicine de Bordeaux, Bordeaux, France.*

A. PYE, *Institute of Laryngology and Otology, London, England.*

T. S. RUSSELL, *The Victoria Infirmary, Glasgow, Scotland.*

S. D. G. STEPHENS, *Institute of Sound and Vibration Research, University of Southampton, Southampton, England.*

I. A. STEWART, *Department of Otolaryngology, University of Dundee, Dundee, Scotland.*

I. G. TAYLOR, *Department of Audiology and Education of the Deaf, The University, Manchester, England.*

W. TAYLOR, *Department of Social and Occupational Medicine, University of Dundee, Dundee, Scotland.*

W. TEMPEST, *Department of Electrical Engineering, University of Salford, Salford, England.*

J. W. TEMPLER, *Central Institute for the Deaf, St. Louis, Missouri, U.S.A.*

I. C. WHITFIELD, *Neurocommunications Research Unit, University of Birmingham, England.*

* Now at Dorval, P. Q., Canada

Foreword

Since its formation, the British Society of Audiology has shown a surprisingly rapid rate of growth, with a membership now standing at over 400. This is but one index of the interest, in Britain, in hearing and its disorders, a subject which concerns people of diverse callings, including those in education, in medicine and in science.

Encouraged by this growing interest in audiology, the Council of the British Society of Audiology decided to inaugurate a series of four-yearly conferences to be held in association with the British Academic Conferences in Otolaryngology, with which subject many aspects of audiology are related. Support for the First Conference, of which this book is a record, vindicated our belief that such a conference was timely and more than justified the efforts of the Congress President, Dr William Taylor, and his Organizing Committee to ensure that the Conference would be a success.

Ronald Hinchcliffe *April 1973*

Preface

This volume contains the full text of papers presented at the First British Conference of the British Society of Audiology, held in the University of Dundee from 14th to 16th July, 1971. The University of Dundee has been honoured by being chosen by the Council of the British Society of Audiology as the organizers of the First of four-yearly conferences planned in association with the British Conferences in otolaryngology.

In planning the Conference the organizers took the opportunity of commemorating one of the outstanding pioneers and a key-founder of audiology—Dr Thomas Simm Littler—by initiating "The Thomas Simm Littler Memorial Lecture".

The Council wish to express their grateful thanks to Sir Alexander Ewing for delivering this inaugural lecture at our British Society's First Conference and this memorial lecture is reproduced in this volume in full. The contribution to audiology made by Dr Littler has also been commemorated by an annual award for the most outstanding research work done in the previous year. The opportunity was taken at the Conference to present this award to Dr John Bench, Reading.

The papers read at the Conference, and collected in this volume, cover a wide field, the deliberate aim of the organizers being to appeal not only to experts and research workers but to all those concerned clinically with the measurement of hearing. Although the academic and clinical departments in Dundee have been mainly concerned with noise-induced hearing loss, this is but one aspect of the growing world-wide interest in noise measurement, in the reduction of noise both in industry and in the community, and in the measurement of hearing loss by subjective and objective methods. Audiology has now been firmly established in such widely diversified areas as industry, hospitals, schools and universities. Thus the papers presented in this volume reflect the interests of many people in many disciplines—in medicine, in science and in education.

The Editor would like to record the help received in organizing the Conference from the President of the Society, Dr R. Hinchcliffe and from Mrs W. M. Massie, the Conference Secretary, the latter serving in many varied roles before, during and after the Conference. The organizers would like also to express their grateful thanks to Mr R. P. Itter, Secretary to the British Society of Audiology and to the Chairmen of sessions.

W. Taylor   *April 1973*
University of Dundee

Contents

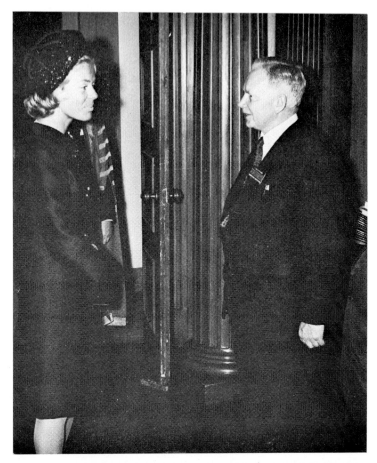

Dr Thomas Simm Littler, Ph.D., F.Inst.P., with H.R.H. The
Duchess of Kent at the IX International Congress of Audiology held
in London in 1968.

One of the key founders of Audiology, it is very fitting that Dr T. S.
Littler was commemorated at the British Society's First Conference.
Beginning at Manchester University in 1933, he pioneered electronic
hearing aids for the hard of hearing and broad-band amplification for
deaf children. After being a Senior Scientific Officer in the Royal Air
Force during World War II and Senior Lecturer in Acoustics at
Manchester, he was appointed in 1949, by the Medical Research
Council, as Director of its newly established Wernher Research Unit
on Deafness. He made notable contributions in research on noise-
induced hearing loss and presbyacusis. Amongst his staff and collaborators were W. Burns, T. E. Cawthorne, R. R. A. Coles, R.
Hinchcliffe, J. J. Knight, C. G. Rice and D. W. Robinson. From the
Royal Society of Medicine he was awarded in 1951, its Norman
Gamble Prize for the most outstanding contributions in Otology
in the preceding five years. Notable among his many writings was
his book "The Physics of the Ear", published in 1965.

The Thomas Simm Littler Memorial Lecture

The Place and Functions of Audiology in the Community

SIR ALEXANDER EWING

Alderley Edge, Cheshire, England

This lecture celebrates the memory of Thomas Simm Littler. I am deeply grateful for the honour and privilege of having been invited to give it.

Dr Littler was one of the pioneer founders of audiology. His personal researches, his many contributions to the relevant professional journals, and lectures to most of the appropriate societies and institutions, together with his book *The Physics of the Ear* published in 1965, have assured him an international reputation. Of equally outstanding value to our community was his constant and continuing service to governmental authorities in peace and war. He will always be an outstanding figure, in the history of audiology. Yet he never sought honours. Speaking as a collaborator and a friend, I will say he played an essential part in the development of the Manchester University Department and in the shaping of my own career. Later, I will refer to some aspects of his work and thinking, particularly as regards communication.

Audiology is a convergence of disciplines comparable to a junction at which a number of roads meet. This is well summarized by Hayes Newby in the first edition of his book *Audiology*.

> If the mother and father of audiology are speech pathology and otology then . . . among the medical relatives are pediatrics, gerontology, psychiatry and neurology. Pediatricians and gerontologists represent extremes in ages of patients, yet both are concerned with problems of impaired hearing as they affect the health and adjustment of their patients.

He went on to refer to maladjustments, frequently caused by hearing impairments, auditory disorders involving pathology of the nervous system, clinical psychologists as an important unit in the team approach and of course to acoustics and electronics. He described audiology as

> related to education, particularly in matters concerning the training of deaf and hard of hearing children.

Under this heading in the field of paedo-audiology, he emphasized the necessity of a specialized knowledge of the principles and practice of training pre-school and school-age children, and close co-operation with teachers. It is no wonder that at the end of this chapter Newby concluded

> No one individual can be expected to be the complete audiologist.

We might also state that audiology is a field in which great advances, in many directions, have been made in the last four decades. The subjects included in the index to Volumes 1–9 of the journal *International Audiology*, 1962–70, are classified under 54 headings. As a profession we are concerned with auditory stimulation, auditory sensation and what might be described as auditory de-sensitization, and both with sound wanted and sound unwanted.

Audiology began and developed primarily as a "humane science". These two words describe essential features of the personality of T. S. Littler. When I first knew him, 40 years ago, he had resigned his appointment as Senior Lecturer in Physics at the Egyptian University, Cairo, because he wanted opportunities for research, then lacking there. He had driven back to England in his Fiat car, including a drive up Mount Vesuvius as part of his itinerary! Running repairs to cars were always well within his scope. On one occasion, in the centre of Manchester, he diagnosed a car break-down as due to a fault in the ignition distributor, then repaired it with the graphite core of a "lead" pencil. Another time, halted on a trans-Pennine road journey by fracture of the transmission shaft, the local garage owner could not undertake to repair his car. Within a few hours Littler had himself obtained and fitted the necessary spare part.

When he returned from Egypt Tom Littler's potential value to research on human pathologies was quickly perceived by our then Reader in Human Physiology, F. W. Lamb. It was while he was investigating detection and measurement of heart murmurs by electronic techniques that Dr Lamb brought him to see us. Tom Littler was motivated to begin what became his life-long work because he realized that deafness results in specific human needs. Within three years he pioneered the valve-amplifying group hearing aids for use in special schools that our previous data had shown to be urgently needed. They were constructed to his own design in our University Department.

Confronted with the problems of severe deafness in hard of hearing adults he quickly conceived the idea several years before 1939, that electronic hearing aids should be made available to all who needed them and he arranged with an electrical engineering firm to produce a small portable aid at low cost—the progenitor, of course, of our British National Health Service hearing aids.

To the end of his life Dr Littler saw the prosthetic requirements of hearing-impaired people as a vital function of audiology in its service to the community. In our excellent journal *Sound* (initiated and edited by him) he wrote, within eighteen months of his death (Littler, 1968), a short article "Can alleviation by hearing aids be improved?" I will discuss later what I believe may be the fundamental importance of his discussion in that article. Earlier in the 1960s he had already made an important contribution towards better alleviation by hearing aids for deaf children. His survey for the London County Council Committee on "Improved Hearing Aid Equipment" related to data showing that there is a considerable incidence of better capacity for response to sound of low than of high frequencies among children diagnosed as severely or profoundly deaf. With typical ingenuity Littler adapted the Medresco OL.58 bone conduction hearing aid for use with a modified air conduction receiver. This, as many of you may know, enabled a much smoother low-frequency performance to be obtained as compared with the Medresco OL.57, when fitted with a 575 receiver. In his report Littler stated that severely deaf children, without exception, preferred the modified OL.58 aid to the OL.57. His finding has been followed up by production of a new aid but not yet, I understand, available for the benefit of all deaf children when supplied with hearing aids through our National Health Service.

This finding marks a step forward towards some effective and practical conclusions about the long-controverted problem of selective prescription of hearing aids. In Littler's own words

> . . . it was felt that more efficient use could be made of the Medresco aid . . . by providing a testing service where the response characteristics of each aid could be obtained, and in consequence allocating those aids with higher gain and outputs to the more severely deaf children and the wider frequency responses to those who would benefit most by their use. . . . It is again suggested that the Committee should seriously consider that an issuing and testing centre be created with the service of the L.C.C. schools.

Embodied in these last statements, therefore, we have recommendations firstly for audiologists selectively to prescribe a type of hearing aid specifically designed to suit an aural condition that it is for them to take steps to identify—and secondly for the performance of each hearing aid of a particular design (in Littler's report the Medresco) to be evaluated—say with the Brüel and Kjaer apparatus—in order that an audiologist might know it to be capable of meeting an individual patient's need. Successive investigations of particular types of hearing aid in the Manchester University laboratories in my time as Director and since have confirmed the validity of the second point.

That certain identifiable groups of hearing-aid users do best with hearing aids designed to provide specific performances in terms of frequency bands was also reported by Dr A. M. Boothroyd at the Mexico Congress and in *International Audiology* (Boothroyd, 1967). His tests were given to 25 children aged 8 to 15 years, all of them pupils in a school for the partially hearing, diagnosed as having perceptive hearing losses. In the following year Dr Daniel Ling of McGill University and Mrs Doris Leckie of the Montreal Oral School for the Deaf reported that they had tackled this problem with 12 children who had residual hearing mainly restricted to low frequencies. They stated that, with a standard model hearing aid amplifying from 250 Hz to 3 kHz, the vowel /ee/ was audible only up to about 3 ft, although they could hear the vowel /ah/ at 30 ft. With one of the more recently developed type of body-worn aids (amplifying from 100 Hz to 3 kHz) all vowels and voiced consonants were audible to all the twelve children at 35–40 ft. I myself have obtained somewhat similar results. For every patient, surely, the first function of a hearing aid is that it should make as much as possible of the speech area available to him.

As regards very profoundly deaf children I believe that Dr A. M. Boothroyd's report at last year's Stockholm Congress has great significance. Defining this category of children as those

> ... who have no response to sound within the standard audiometric range or who respond at low frequencies only and within or close to the range of tactile sensitivity

he stated that in experiments with classroom equipment at the Clarke School, Massachusetts, where he is now Director of Research, he has found that

> ... the first requirement for such children is a good low frequency response extending at least as far as 100 Hz.

To introduce my next point I should like to quote the final sentence in Dr Littler's editorial article on improvement of alleviation by hearing aids to which I have already referred. After stating that

> ... for the majority of deaf subjects a form of wide-band frequency response that is smooth in character has been confirmed over and over again as the most satisfactory.

He refers to the finding that binaural hearing, so far, does not seem

to have produced anything like the striking results so helpful to normals . . .

Then he asks what I believe to be a key question

—Is it not now appropriate that we should review the whole field to see if we should do some re-thinking of the situation?

He questions whether the partial failure of prosthetic provision of binaural hearing is related to

. . . the need for special training in binaural reception for deaf ears which have not experienced this faculty.

I would strongly urge that this subject of special training is worthy of far more research by audiologists than it has ever yet received. As regards use of binaural amplification through two separate electronic channels, with their separate microphones picking up sound at two separate points in space, our observation is that there may be hard of hearing patients who can achieve directional hearing with two ear-level hearing aids. Is it not possible that, as Littler has asked, some subjects could achieve the same invaluable ability, as a result of training and with adequate amplification, in spite of never having enjoyed it before in their lives? I am thinking of both children and adults with a diagnosis of life-long sensori-neural deafness. Of course, one has worked with the experienced hearing-aid user in this category who reports that

What I hear in this ear sounds quite different from what I hear in the other ear

but this does not apply to all patients.

The problem of achieving directional hearing in particular cases may or may not be insurmountable. It may well be so, for instance, when causation is diagnosed as retrocochlear, with a sub-cortical or cortical pathology seriously affecting the neurological mechanism of hearing. This would be implied, for example, by Jeffress (1971).

The practical issue is surely that even if only a minority of hearing aid wearers could be given ability to use directional cues this would help them to cope with one of the most severe forms of difficulty which they constantly encounter—namely discriminating speech signals against a background of noise and reverberation. Recently, I myself experienced deprivation of binaural hearing for some weeks. This confirmed most conclusively a sentence in my wife's and my book (Ewing and Ewing, 1964), namely that

binaural hearing is also known to affect very significantly capacity to listen discriminately to sound from a particular source in conditions in which reverberation and noise are present.

In the same passage we noted that our former colleague at Manchester University, J. E. J. John, had pointed out that listening to speech in a traditional type of school classroom (hard plaster walls, etc.) is made much more difficult for a normally hearing person if he plugs one ear tightly with a finger and that he will be particularly conscious of the improvement when he unplugs that ear. My own experiment was prolonged as well as unplanned! There was no difficulty about speech reception in our own quiet home with plenty of soft furnishings. In conversations before and after a crowded public meeting, or even in a shop with plenty of noise present, the difficulty was great. There is abundance of evidence that this whole problem of listening to speech in a noise is acute for many thousands of school children, when they are supplied with a single hearing aid, on which they must rely for much of their education, when placed in ordinary schools with non-sound-treated classrooms. As contrasted with how they hear in a sound-treated clinic, the accuracy with which they hear speech is halved.

Returning to Dr Littler's point about the probability of a need for special training in binaural reception for deaf ears which have not previously experienced it, the word "inhibition" comes to mind in this context. It was described by Professor Von Békésy of Harvard in 1960 as a factor in selective listening. For instance

> at a social gathering when several people are talking simultaneously we can concentrate our attention on a single speaker and suppress all the others to a certain degree.

Here we are confronted with a function of the nervous system. Beginning in infancy, we start to learn to identify sound patterns and sources of sound and to rotate head and eyes in its direction is a very important aid in the early stages of this learning process, as my wife and I have seen illustrated in tests of the hearing of hundreds of infants found to have unimpaired hearing. (For a valuable review of neurological mechanisms of hearing, see Hawkins, 1964.)

It would certainly seem that the whole subject of learning, as a means of developing what Tom Littler called improvement of alleviation by hearing aids, requires much more attention and, indeed, research by audiologists. In a recent article the Principal of the Mary Hare Grammar School, R. Askew, has described practical means of meeting some of the difficulties encountered by former pupils successful in qualifying for admission to universities (Askew, 1971). In an experiment, in 1969, radio-microphone transmitters were handed to lecturers and radio-hearing aids to students, three of whom were described as partially hearing rather than partially deaf. They were rejected by the students. By contaast, during the past year prolonged training in the use of these aids, with present senior pupils in the school, suggests that they may be willing to take the instruments with them and use them when they enter universities. It might be suggested also that some guidance to the lecturers involved would be helpful as regards microphone techniques, particularly if the microphones are at all directional.

In the same journal is an article on "Hearing Impaired Children in Ordinary Schools". The author is the County Organizer of the Service for Children with Impaired Hearing (educational psychologist) Lancashire County Council, Brian Fisher. He states (Fisher, 1971) that in a personal study of 83 children with impaired hearing, attending ordinary classes, mean hearing loss 38 decibels, he found considerable retardation in attainments and significantly poor emotional and social adjustment. Referring back to the substantial study by Reeves (1961), of pupils with impaired hearing in ordinary schools, Fisher says that Reeves' results "strongly underline the need for guidance in the use of hearing aids by these children . . .". Surely, training as well as guidance is necessary for most or all of those children! My experience, and that of my wife, in recent years, at local authority audiology clinics, has been that not a few children, supplied with hearing aids and certainly need-ing amplification, had clearly discarded them. Relevant at this point is an experience at this year's annual conference of the British Association of the Hard of Hearing when I heard statements that a good many adults supplied with hearing aids keep them "on the shelf".

For children, aural habilitation may be a better term than aural rehabilitation. There is also the subject of development of auditory discrimination. Wepman (1960) found that in the condition of unim-paired hearing the development of auditory discrimination continues to progress up to the age of 8 years. In home training and educational treatment of children with defective hearing it proceeds more slowly. Verbal development clearly continues far longer in the lives of indi-viduals. It has been well said that for children new words and linguistic forms constitute nonsense words until they have acquired meaning.

I would strongly urge that a new concept and definition of the term "socially adequate" as applied to children whose hearing is impaired needs to be provided by paedo-audiologists. Always in the back of my mind, in this connection, is the report by Fletcher (1929). Giving very extensive data on the significance of frequency bands to the intelligibility of heard speech, he stated that nonsense syllables had proved the most searching form of test material, but that their Bell Laboratory research teams needed about two weeks' practice before reliable results were obtained in particular conditions.

I presume that all audiologists would agree with Brian Fisher's criticism that the rough types of speech tests used by parents, teachers and doctors, consisting as they do usually of familiar words, are likely to pass the child as socially adequate but the criterion is clearly inadequate for educational purposes.

He has referred to the accepted finding in speech audiometry that, when only 50 per cent of the individual sounds of speech are heard, the listener can easily understand ordinary connected speech and to the fact that this 50 per cent discrimination level has been considered to indicate socially adequate hearing. I am altogether on Fisher's side in thinking that it is very unlikely that this 50 per cent phonetic discrimination level has similar criterion value for the speech hearing of children. Modern communication theory is greatly increasing and clarifying our under-standing of the extent to which we rely on experience, gradually accumulated, of the phonetic patterning and word and sentence forms typical of any one language to become efficient in receptive and expres-sive use of it. Van Uden (1970) has well demonstrated significance of communication theory in our field.

Children's personality adjustment as well as their development linguistically, socially, intellectually and educationally, have now clearly been found to be affected by problems in communication. And this is not just at school. In attempting to assess the social adequacy of a hearing-impaired child I would suggest consideration of such variables as speaker efficiency, particularly of his parents and of the teachers whom he daily encounters. I will return later to variations in acoustic environment and capacity to cope with them, with special reference to distortions of sound patterns by acoustic imprint.

I have found very interesting a brief, summarized report of a 1970 survey by the Victorian Branch of the Australian Association for Better Hearing. It is based on a questionnaire addressed to current members and to hearing-impaired people who had received help from the Associa-tion within the last few years—number not quoted. People were asked to state their needs in order of importance to themselves. They were requested to place the figures 1, 2, 3, 4, 5 against the headings: lip-reading; speech conservation; hearing re-education; how to get the best results with your hearing aid; social opportunities. The replies showed that communication by lip-reading and hearing was given far higher priority than social opportunities by these hard of hearing adults. Lip-reading came first of all with most of them. Hearing re-education had first priority with 8 per cent and how to get the best results with your hearing aid with 15 per cent. Fifty per cent placed hearing re-education their second priority out of the possible five.

On the basis of personal first-hand experience with both children and adults, I would make suggestions under two headings: firstly recommendation as to the type of aid suitable for the individual patient; secondly, methods of helping patients to get the best results with hearing aids. To provide facilities for these procedures on a national scale a much larger force of audiologists is needed than is at present available. As regards hearing-impaired children in ordinary schools peripatetic teachers of the deaf already co-operate.

RECOMMENDATION AS TO THE TYPE OF HEARING AID SUITABLE FOR THE INDIVIDUAL PATIENT

Surely the first question is to what extent and in what bands of frequency could Hearing Aid X make the speech area available to this patient? I think of the form used in the Manchester University Department of Audiology and Education of the Deaf for marking in results of pure-tone audiometry. Already shaded on the form before use is the area typical of the sound of conversational speech at the 65 decibel level, a distance of 3 ft. The patient's audiogram, when completed, indicates immediately how much of the typical speech area may be made audible to him when listening with each ear, unaided. Next a hearing aid. The expert audiologist with access to performance curves of aids marks on the form the boundaries to which the speech area can reasonably be expected to be extended through amplification. In the United Kingdom one of the existing types of National Health Service Medresco aids is likely to be the audiologist's first choice for many, or most, patients. Already, earlier in this lecture, I have referred to modern research findings that I accept as relevant to selective prescription of aids in certain aural conditions. Local health authorities, for which we have worked, are prepared to pay for commercially supplied hearing aids for children when clearly proved to be necessary.

Next I want to include a test of each ear by standardized speech audiometry—using P.B. lists or modified versions of them for younger school children with more limited vocabularies. Speech audiometry is time consuming but provided that a patient has the necessary vocabulary, or, if a child, is sufficiently mature, its results can indicate so clearly, in most cases, (a) the patient's best hearing potential and (b) his best hearing level—in ideal acoustic conditions. Where deafness has particularly impaired hearing in the upper frequency part of the speech area, relevant types of consonantal error afford a significant indication of this.

Next, if the scale of staffing that is really very necessary is available I would make a first try-out with the hearing aid so far indicated as most appropriate and likely to be most beneficial to the individual patient. The try-out to be made in the sound-treated clinic to explore informally, as a first step, how closely, in the patient's present auditory state, the degree of accuracy with which the selected hearing aid enables him to follow speech matches up to his hearing potential as revealed by speech audiometry. Informality at this stage makes possible a quick change to trial with an alternative type of aid if the first choice seems to be questioned by new evidence. I should use a method of monitored live voice at least at two distances, 3 ft and at 9 ft. Different aspects of the problem of supplying efficient ear-moulds are too familiar for me to discuss here.

METHODS OF HELPING PATIENTS TO GET THE BEST RESULTS WITH HEARING AIDS

In the clinic, when a patient is first supplied with a recommended hearing aid, the audiologist shows him how he is adjusting volume control and, if included, tone control, to obtain best results in the trial so far made. A little practice in adjusting the volume control, if necessary, to speech at different levels of loudness, can be useful. Presence or absence of recruitment is a factor which is investigated under the heading of diagnostic procedures, in the audiologist's co-operation with an otolaryngologist to which I will refer later. As regards hearing aid usage the practical point, of course, is to find by testing, particularly in the case of children when unable to find out for themselves, the narrow range of volume settings within which the patient's tolerance for amplification and efficient hearing is available. That this is necessary for a good many children has been conclusively indicated by the researches of Harold (1957) and others.

My main point here is that initial supply of a hearing aid is only a first step. Improvement of alleviation by hearing aids for very many patients is essentially dependent on provision of a follow-up service. I am credibly informed from various sources that such a follow-up service is not yet available in the case of a good many adult patients but that it would be welcomed by them.

It is not just a patient's capacity for speech reception in the clinic that is in question but, far more important, his ability to benefit from hearing-aid use, helped out when possible by lip-reading, in real life conditions. Peripatetic teachers, responsible for hearing-impaired children in ordinary schools, whom we have known, are accustomed to the need of assessing acoustic conditions in different schools, with an eye to selective school placement when practicable, and guidance to teachers about classroom positioning and the value of facility for lip-reading. It is on this pattern that a comprehensive follow-up service, for children and for hard of hearing adults, is required.

As regards children I do not think it necessary here to discuss allocation of responsibilities under different forms of authority. A major reorganization is already in progress, both of medical and social services, with the object of securing closer co-operation between different categories of workers. What are the necessities under the heading of audiology? There is a need not only for a child himself to accept use of a hearing aid, when prescribed, but also for his parents to do so. Demonstration can be the first step, beginning by showing them how much more the child can hear with the aid than without it. It can be a great help to interpret in non-technical terms the information provided by the child's audiogram, when marked in on the diagram that includes the typical speech area. Sceptical parents, we have found, can often be converted by hearing a tape recording of filtered speech. We report in detail, in our 1971 book, methods of involving pre-school age children in co-operative play with selected materials, to motivate them to enjoy use of hearing aids. It is just about vital that, whatever a child's age, if he needs a hearing aid, his parents and he shall come to realize it as an effective means of satisfactory communication between them.

With all severely deaf children who have never heard normally there is surely a need to provide training, over a long period, with all the day-by-day auditory experience necessary for them, neurologically and mentally, to develop auditory discrimination and capacity to identify sources of sound. Audiologists will be aware that in deaf as well as in children with unimpaired hearing, these abilities are best developed during the first five years of life when it is normal for children to be making ever-increasing contact with their environment. Expert remedial teaching, in recent decades, has demonstrated the value of developing auditory discrimination in children even when capacity for it is severely limited by aural pathology.

All this emphasizes the conclusion, widely accepted, that parents as well as teachers, need to acquire the relevant special skills. This surely applies to all families in which there is a child with an auditory defect or an auditory disorder. Microphone techniques are skills in which audiologists are particularly well qualified to give guidance and practice. For many children whose hearing is defective there are two requisites. The first is that they need the best performance of which their hearing aids are capable. The variations in levels of loudness that are often evident in the mean loudness levels of casual speech fail to ensure this. We have found that some parents, in individual sessions, have been helped by practice with loudness level meters. Where speech or auditory training units are in use their output metres are very handy for this purpose. Rate of speaking often needs a good deal of attention. The whole point is that, in terms of communication theory, the children need every auditory cue, that can possibly be beneficial to them, clearly presented. This applies, also, to lip-reading.

A technological problem to which I would urgently beg audiologists to give their attention is provision, for severely deaf children, of an effective ear to voice link. Again and again, my wife and I have seen that, when severely deaf children have learnt to realize that through amplification they could hear their own voices, this has become an important part of their lives. I always think, in this connection, of one of my wife's very deaf pupils, at the age of 7, reading to herself, at every opportunity and entirely on her own initiative, with an auditory and speech training unit. The practical point is that children, like this one, need to hear their own voices whenever they speak, at all times. How far, for a majority of them, is this possible with their present body-worn or ear-level hearing aids? I am quite certain that this is an urgent subject for research.

Another subject which I would commend as particularly urgent for research in audiology is to find means of reducing to a minimum the acoustic imprint. This is a subject of great significance, in modern, real life situations, to many hard of hearing adults as well as to hearing-impaired children: but to the children most of all. It is surely no exaggeration to say that not only are the children learning their communication skills in the face of the handicap of deafness but that also they are very unlikely ever to experience again, in their lives, such loud and clear speech signals as may be provided for them in schools, by specially trained staff, with good equipment. There is plenty of experimental data to show the extent to which typical room noise and reverberation, in untreated school classrooms, reduces speech intelligibility to users of body-worn or ear-level hearing aids. Spectrographic analysis makes only too clear the distortion that is involved as regards the sound patterning of speech. Tape recordings of speech in noise through hearing aids demonstrate the problem dramatically to listeners with unimpaired hearing. (Incidentally, from some tentative experiments with tape recordings that I suggested it would seem possible that clear speech from a woman with a good voice emerges from the noise with more clarity than a man's.)

The signal to noise and room reverberation ratio is held at its best, in special schools and units for the deaf and partially hearing, when group hearing aids are expertly used by teachers and pupils. As long as each pupil is provided with a microphone, either swan-neck or cheek microphone, the ear to voice link and pupil–pupil communication (which is just as important as teacher–pupil communication) can be effectively maintained.

A current break-through, enormously facilitating communication for very deaf children, is one that my wife and I have very recently been privileged to see demonstrated. This is regular and constant use of closed-circuit television in combination with sound amplification. This is scientifically planned and most expertly used by the Headmaster, Mr Sam Blount, and his staff at the Nutfield Priory Secondary School for the Deaf, Surrey Education Authority. Since 1968 it has been applied in school assemblies, classroom teaching and individual speech training. I believe that, as audiologists, we are concerned with all means of improving direct personal communication through the spoken word. The multiplication of cues through the screen—enlarged faces of speakers, synchronized with amplification of their utterances, often using inductance systems, brings a new vitality to school life. At the Institute for the Deaf, Sint Michielsgestel, Holland, we saw, in 1969, closed-circuit television brought into action in remedial education for children with special communication problems. Video-tape recordings and replays to individual pupils of themselves speaking were part of the technique.

Radio microphones and radio receivers, body-worn, evidently offer a favourable signal to noise ratio. I have not yet had an opportunity of seeing them used by hearing-impaired children but have read very promising reports of their introduction into certain schools for the deaf.

Referring again to Dr Hayes Newby's comprehensive summary of the functions of audiologists and his reference to co-operation with teachers of the deaf: I hope that some of our colleagues will give their specialized and expert assistance in exploitation for deaf children of continuing technological advances.

AUDIOLOGICAL SERVICES FOR HARD OF HEARING ADULTS

The new organization of medical and social provision, to cover all the handicapped who need it, now being planned in the United Kingdom, should include Area Communication Advisers. Trained in audiology and perhaps in social work also—but with audiology as their essential priority —they would provide a follow-up service for all hard of hearing adults.

When Tom Littler had made his pioneer, valve-amplifying hearing aids available, at a low price, in the 1930s we held weekly hearing-aid sessions at Manchester University for medically referred patients. The link between those sessions and the evening classes that we held for hard of hearing adults was very close. Later, in post-war years, my own methodology for them developed to include graduated training of which the first stage was practice with a wide-band group hearing aid, listening supplemented by watching. The patients thus had opportunity to explore for themselves their best listening levels, and indeed their hearing potentials, in unstressed conditions. (Naturally, I monitored the loudness level of my speech.) In later stages there was practice with their individual hearing aids in reception of each other's speech and, necessarily, I believe, practice in lip-reading without the help of amplification.

The functions of my Area Communication Advisers would include a similar programme, based on Hearing Aid Centres and Clubs for the Hard of Hearing within the area. "How to get the best help from a hearing aid" can be immensely facilitated by guidance and help to husbands and wives, other relatives with whom a hard of hearing patient is in frequent contact, and friends, in the good microphone techniques and speech really clear for lip-reading to which I have already referred. In an area of the extent now contemplated there will surely be need for one or more full-time Communication Advisers, once their availability and the scope of the help that they can give is adequately publicized. An essential part of the adviser's programme would be home visits, particularly to patients prevented from attendance at clinics or clubs by ill-health or age.

Close contact with the British Association of the Hard of Hearing emphasizes the statistical fact that a very large proportion of our hard of hearing population consists of over-sixties. Two papers on hearing aids in presbyacusis, given at the London Congress (Niemeyer, 1969; Bentzen et al., 1969) seemed to me admirable. Dr Niemeyer of Marburg stated that cases of presbyacusis with a bradyacusia

> constitute an ever-increasing proportion of the patients of audiological centres, and they are the proper and real problem-patients for the audiological practitioner.

In relation to what I have called acoustic imprint Niemeyer said that the safest way to eliminate surrounding noise, so disturbing to old-age patients, is to use the induction coil. Reading this reminded me that Tom Littler fitted the dining-table of a famous man with inductance a good many years ago. Niemeyer's paper is full of clinically significant findings.

The paper by Bentzen et al., from the Aarhus, Denmark, Hearing Centre states that of 840 patients, seen in three months, 62·6 per cent were over the age of 65. The tabulated statistics of Bentzen et al. are very promising and appear to justify supply of binaural aids after adequate audiological examination. They quote 7,000 patients as having had binaural aids prescribed at their centre. Nevertheless, they conclude

> Our experiences of this treatment emphasize the importance of an intensified effort by the hearing therapists

and on that note I will end.

REFERENCES

Askew, R. (1971). Opportunities for continued education of the deaf in the United Kingdom, *Teacher of the Deaf*, **69**, 407, 175–181.

Bentzen, O., Frost, E. and Skaftason, S. (1969). Treatment with binaural hearing aids in presbyacusis, *Int. Audiol.*, **8**, 4, 529–534.

Boothroyd, A. M. (1967). The discrimination by partially-hearing children of frequency distorted speech, *Int. Audiol.*, **6**, 2, 136–145.

Ewing, A. W. G. and Ewing, E. C. (1964). "Teaching Deaf Children to Talk", Manchester University Press.

Fisher, B. (1971). Hearing-impaired children in ordinary schools, *Teacher of the Deaf*, **69**, 407, 161–174.

Fletcher, H. (1929). "Speech and Hearing", Macmillan, London.

Harold, B. B. (1957). "The effects of variations in intensity on the capacity of deaf children and adults to hear speech with hearing aids", unpublished P.D. thesis, Manchester University Library.

Hawkins, J. E. (1964). *Hearing, A. Rev. Physiol.*, **26**, 453–480.

Jeffress, L. A. (1971). Detection and lateralization of binaural signals, *Audiology*, **10**, 2, 77–84.

Littler, T. S. (1965). "The Physics of the Ear", Pergamon Press, London.

Littler, T. S. (1968). Can alleviation by hearing aids be improved?, *Sound*, **2**, 2, 30.

Newby, H. (1959). "Audiology", Vision Press, London.

Niemeyer, W. (1969). Difficulties and effectivity of hearing aid equipment in presbyacusis, *Int. Audiol.*, **8**, 535–545.

Reeves, J. K. (1961). The use of hearing aids by children with defective hearing, *Teacher of the Deaf*, **59**, 352, 181–190.

Van Uden, A. (1970). "A World of Language for Deaf Children. A Maternal Reflective Method", Rotterdam University Press.

Von Bekesy, G. (1960). "Experiments in Hearing", McGraw-Hill, London, New York.

Wepman, J. M. (1960). Outline of auditory discrimination theory, *Elementary Schools' Journal*, **60**, 325–333.

Aspects of the Aetiology of Deafness

BENGT BARR

Department of Audiology, Karolinska, Sjukhuset,
Stockholm, Sweden

It has hitherto been extremely difficult to identify the cause of deafness in individual children. The aetiological classification of deafness is made on the basis of the medico-audiologic examination and the history, and especially the family history. The information relating to deaf relatives must be weighed against any potentially exogenous factors that might be considered to have a bearing on the child's hearing before, during or after birth, and against the objective findings of the examination. In some cases a hereditary background is so obvious that the hearing defect may be confidently ascribed to an endogenous cause. Often, however, no explanation for the hearing impairment can be found, and the case must then be assigned to the "unknown" group; but there is every reason to suppose that in this group, too, the hearing defect will usually have a genetic origin. In short, the consensus is that the hereditary group comprises about one half of all the child cases of severe hearing impairment. In this group the recessive mode of inheritance is by far the most common.

There are no biochemical tests by which one can detect any abnormal activity of enzymes responsible for the normal structure and function of the auditory system. For this reason it has not been possible to class hereditary deafness as an inborn error of metabolism; but this does not rule out the possibility that it does in fact belong to this group; it means only that our knowledge of the enzymatic action involved in this biological process is still too limited to enable us to ascertain a possible biochemical basis of these defects.

There remains the possibility of detecting the effect of any enzymatic defects on the hearing organ in gene carriers through audiometric examination. The application of common tone-audiometry to disclose as heterozygotes the normal parents of children with hearing impairment has proved unsuccessful. It may thus be assumed that any defects in the heterozygotes are sub-clinical, and that to obtain a solution of the problem more sensitive tests than have been used so far must be applied.

One such test is provided by Békésy audiometry, where by the continuous recording of the hearing threshold even quite small deviations can be detected. Another possibility is to determine the threshold for the stapedius reflex, a method that also has the merit of objectivity.

GENETIC STIGMATA IN HEARING THRESHOLD

The series for the investigation comprised 30 pairs of parents with subjectively normal hearing, and 74 children, 48 of whom had severe hereditary hearing impairment. The genetic taint is confirmed by the fact that no less than 15 of the families had two or more children with impaired hearing. In 12 of the families there was also information on other relatives with probably endogenous deafness.

In some of the parents Békésy disclosed sharply demarcated threshold increases in the range 250–3,000 Hz (dips) in an otherwise normal threshold. These dips were regarded as significant if they attained at least 20 dB hearing level, extended over at least one octave and reached at least 6 dB at the limits of this frequency range. Such dips (Fig. 1 were recorded for three of the fathers (10 per cent) and seven of the mothers (23 per cent).

To be able to decide whether a certain peculiarity in otherwise

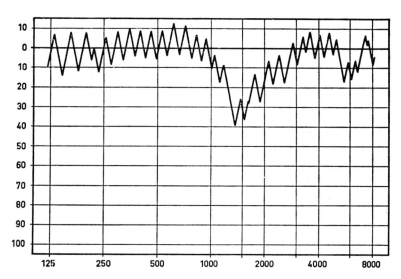

FIG. 1. Example of dip in hearing threshold recorded by Békésy audiometry. Note that its frequency is such that the dip might be missed in routine octave audiometry.

normal hearing might be considered as an endogenous stigma it is necessary to know its degree and frequency of occurrence in an average group. Békésy audiometry in a control group of 60 women and 73 men disclosed this peculiarly in only 1·5 per cent; such dips would thus seem to be extremely rare among normals. This has since been confirmed by other workers in larger series of normals.

In contrast to impairments in the high-frequency range the mid-frequency dips and basins have no known exogenous cause. This, together with the frequent occurrence of dips in the hereditary series, points to a genetic origin; support for this is found in the fact that the

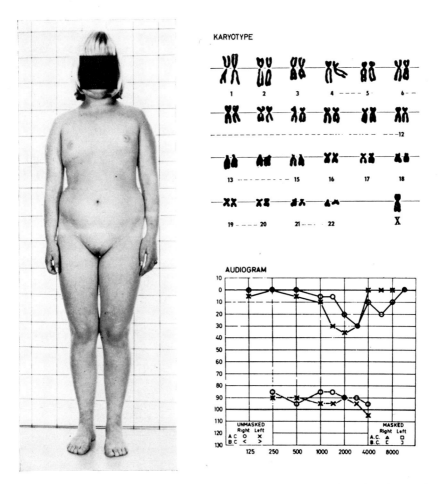

FIG. 2. A case of Turner's syndrome (short stature, ovarian dysgenesis and various mal-formations in females having structural abnormalities of the X chromosome). The octave audiogram shows the typical threshold dip.

same type of mid-frequency dips is found in Turner's syndrome, a typical genetic disease. The underlying cause here is a sex chromosome aberration (Fig. 2). We have found the same type of mid-frequency dips is not less than 42 per cent of 75 Turner cases examined at Karolinska Hospital.

GENETIC STIGMATA IN STAPEDIUS REFLEX THRESHOLD

It is known from previous studies that the reflex threshold in the frequency range 250–4,000 Hz normally lies between 80 and 90 dB hearing level for the various test frequencies. The stapedius reflex threshold is extremely resistant to exogenous agents such as noise, antibiotics, etc. Even persons where years of exposure to noise combined with presbyacusis have given rise to considerable elevation of the hearing thresholds still may record reflex thresholds within normal limits.

Only a few conditions are known where abnormal elevation of the reflex threshold results from exogenous or known agents; with extremely rare exceptions there is simultaneous elevation of the hearing threshold, and the overall audiometric pattern in these cases is that of a retrocochlear impairment.

Occasionally, however, persons are encountered with completely normal hearing function in all respects but whose reflex thresholds are

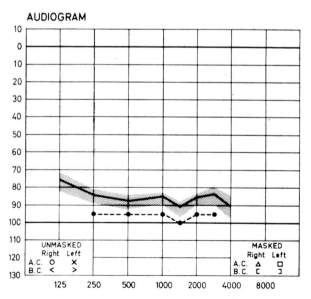

FIG. 3. Median and semi-interquartile range (shaded) for reflex threshold of the 200 ears of the control group. . – – – – . – – – – . The lower limit for pathologic threshold values.

elevated without any obvious exogenous explanation. To determine the occurrence of subjects with elevated reflex thresholds in spite of completely normal hearing thresholds a study was performed with the aim also to specify at which level a reflex threshold should be regarded as abnormally high.

The means and ranges of the reflex threshold obtained for 200 normal ears are given in Fig. 3. On the basis of these values a criterion for the pathologic limit was formulated; the boundary is denoted in the figure by the broken line. Only 3 per cent of the subjects with normal hearing recorded reflex thresholds above the limit.

Of the 30 pairs comprising the genetic series only a few parents fell within the normal range. The stapedius thresholds were considerably elevated and at many points could not be reached, even though the hearing thresholds of the subjects almost invariably lay within the normal range (Fig. 4). This condition is illustrated most strikingly in

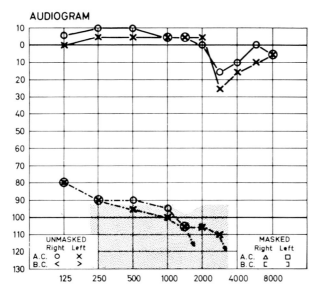

FIG. 4. Hearing and reflex thresholds for a case in the hereditary group. The values within the shaded area lie above the pathologic limit.

the youngest ears where the hearing threshold still did not display any signs of exogenous impairment (Fig. 5).

The hereditary group thus showed a vast over-representation of elevated reflex thresholds (Fig. 6). In view of the hereditary taint of the group and the absence of any known exogenous explanation of this specific defect it would seem reasonable to conclude that this anomaly is

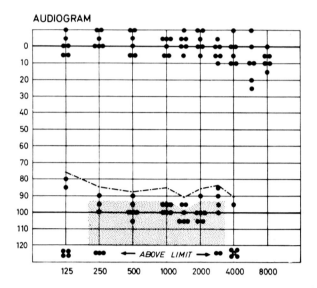

FIG. 5. Hearing and reflex thresholds for the six youngest ears in the hereditary group that fell for the reflex criterion. . − . − . − . Median of the control group. The values within the shaded area lie above the pathologic limit.

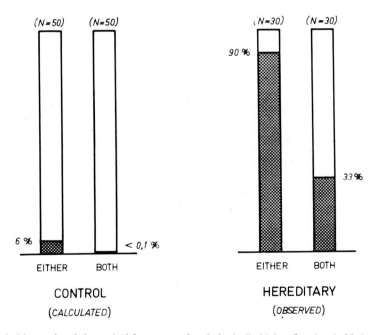

FIG. 6. Observed and theoretical frequency of pathologically high reflex thresholds in one or both marriage partners.

of genetic origin. Support for this inference is provided by subsequent frequent observations of abnormally high reflex thresholds in a well-defined genetic disorder—Klinefelter's syndrome (Fig. 7).

To summarize: by using two sensitive hearing tests, namely, continuous recording of the hearing threshold by Békésy audiometry and by determination of the stapedius reflex threshold, it seems possible to detect at least one group of carriers of genes for deafness in persons with subjectively normal hearing. The application of this method in parents to deaf children reveals in many cases a hereditary etiology of hearing impairments earlier classified as "unknown".

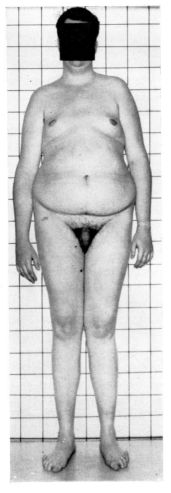

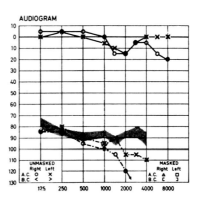

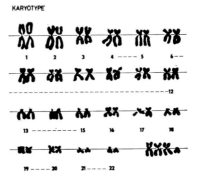

FIG. 7. Hearing and reflex thresholds in a characteristic case of Klinefelter's syndrome (various sex chromosome anomalies). Reflex threshold values are above the pathologic limit.

GENETIC STIGMATA IN MATERNAL RUBELLA DEAFNESS

Rubella infection in the first three to four months of pregnancy incurs a serious risk of damage to the child, the most common manifestations being heart disorders, eye defects, hearing impairments and mental disturbances. The risk figures for this maternal rubella syndrome have been variously reported as between 7 and 23 per cent. The chance of a severe hearing impairment occurring, alone or in combination with other defects, is on the whole relatively small (3 to 8 per cent).

The reason why so remarkably large a proportion of the children display no defects has interested many research workers. The importance of the time for the onset of the infection during pregnancy, the possibility of different types of virus and different immunologic conditions in the mother are among the factors that have been discussed.

Our interest in hereditary hearing disorders led us to consider the possibility of a simultaneous effect of genetic factors. A preliminary survey of the children registered at Karolinska Hospital as having hearing impairments associated with maternal rubella brought to light in many of them a hereditary trait with respect to deafness impairment. This observation prompted a closer examination of the causal connection between a hereditary disposition for hearing impairment and maternal rubella deafness, as the cause of a hearing defect.

The diagnosis of hereditary hearing impairment is based partly on the reported presence of earlier hearing defects in the proband's family. Such information is difficult to evaluate without reference values, and to provide a more reliable basis for an assessment of this factor an analysis was made of the occurrence of hearing impairment in a randomly selected reference group of 500 persons. A questionnaire was distributed containing the same questions relating to the incidence of hearing impairment in the family as were put to the parents of the rubella children.

Over a period of 20 years more than 1,500 children with severe hearing loss or total deafness have been examined at Karolinska Hospital. In 312 of them the hearing defects were ascribed to maternal rubella (Fig. 8). To obtain a representative group suitable for detailed study all such children born in the county of Stockholm during the four-year period 1962–65 were selected. These numbered 20 (including one set of twins) and they and their parents were requested to attend a new examination.

The hearing impairments in the children were confirmed by repeated hearing tests, the method being chosen according to the age and level of development. In all cases the hearing loss was severe enough to call for rehabilitatory measures. Besides the hearing examination, all the

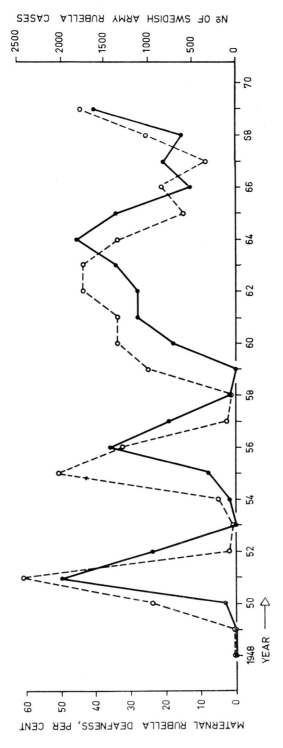

Fig. 8. Comparison of the percentage frequency of maternal rubella deafness registered at the Karolinska Hospital (continuous curve) and the reported number of rubella cases among Swedish army personnel (broken curve) for 1948 to 1969.

children were also submitted to examinations with special regard to the defects typical of maternal rubella. In 17 of the children a haemag-glutination-inhibition and a complement fixation test were performed to detect antibodies of rubella.

On the basis of replies to a questionnaire the time of exposure to rubella, the appearance of clinical symptoms and signs during preg-nancy, the mode of verification, the course of the pregnancy and delivery, and the weight of the child at birth were recorded.

The results of the examinations are given in Table 1. Briefly, there was a remarkably high frequency of defects typical of maternal rubella. Besides characteristic hearing impairment, 16 of the 20 children had at least one other typical anomaly. Furthermore, the fact that a rubella virus infection had occurred was also confirmed by the serologic tests.

The parents were submitted to the usual otologic examination and hearing tests comprising Békésy audiometry and recording of the stapedius reflex. Fourteen of the mothers had the same serologic tests as the children. In addition, a systematic inquiry was made as to the occurrence of endogenous hearing impairments in the parents' families.

The examination disclosed a marked over-representation of here-ditary stigmata in both anamnestic and audiometric findings in the parents.

Out of the 38 parents, 17 knew of hearing impairments in their family of a type ascribable to hereditary factors. This frequency of about 50 per cent is five to ten times greater than that reported for such impairments in the control series, namely 6 per cent. In the parental pairs of these children significant threshold dips were about ten times more common than in the general population. Pathologically high stapedius reflex thresholds were recorded in 13 of the (36) parents or 60 per cent of the parental pairs against 6 per cent of the controls.

Although the evidence points to maternal rubella as being the cause of the deafness, the fact remains that in all 19 families there was also strong evidence of a hereditary trait with respect to hearing impairment. The observations may be taken as an indication of a possible interaction between endogenous (hereditary) and exogenous (rubella virus) factors as cause for the deafness. This might seem a surprising proposition, since maternal rubella has always been considered to be an entirely exogenous cause of hearing loss. A possible explanation is that the genetically deficient organ is more susceptible to the exogenous strain of the virus infection. If this should in fact be the case it would explain why such a large number of children with maternal rubella do not develop hearing defects. From the theoretical standpoint, the observation is a most interesting one in that it is consistent with more recent findings in

Clinical findings in the children with rubella deafness and their parents

							GROUP A												B		C	
Case No.	1	2	3	4a	4b	5	6	7	8	9	10	12	15	16	17	19	13	18	11	14
CHILDREN																				
Hearing loss	+	+	+	+	+	+	+	+	+	+	+	+	+	+	+	+	+	+	+	+
Chorioretinitis			+	+	+	+	+	+				+	+	+	+	+	+	+		+
Cataract	+					+			+							+				
Microphthalmus	+								+											+
Prematurity	+			+	+	+	+					+	+	+			+			
Cong. vitium	+	?				?			+			?				+	+			
Mental retard.	+		+			+			+	+										+
Other defects							+			?					+					+
Seropositive	+	+	+	?	−	+	+	+	+	++	+	−	+	+	+	+	+	+	?	−
PARENTS																				
Heredity	?	+++	+++				+	+	??	+++				?+	+	+		++	++	++
Hearing threshold	?					+		+				++	+	−	+	?+		?+		?
Reflex threshold	?		?+	+++	+++							++	−	−	+		+	+	+	++
Seropositive	−	+	+			−	+	+	−	+	−	−	−	−	−	+	+	+	+	−

Twins (4a, 4b)

Group A: Characteristic symptoms of rubella during pregnancy. Diagnosis verified at physician's examination.
Group B: Exposed during pregnancy, characteristic symptoms present.
Group C: Exposed but no symptoms observed. + Positive finding. ? Questionable finding. − Test not performed.
Blank denotes normal observation. Parent group columns: Mothers = right, Fathers = left.

experimental teratology. The genetic disposition had proved to be a critical factor in the occurrence of malformations from a given teratogen. Between various species and also between various strains of animals there are considerable differences in this respect. It is reasonable to suppose that an interaction of genetic and exogenous factors of this nature that has been demonstrated in animals may also be the cause of teratogenic defects in man. It would, however, seem to be the first time that a connection has been found between a specific genetic defect in an organ and an exogenous agent acting on the same organ—in this case the rubella virus.

SUMMARY

The dominant and sex-linked forms of hereditary hearing loss, which have long been recognized, are readily identified on the basis of the family history and routine hearing tests. The mode of inheritance of the recessive forms of hereditary deafness, on the other hand, has been extremely difficult to identify. Usually, attempts are made to find exogenous factors as the cause of deafness, and where such a "natural" explanation has not been forthcoming the case has been assigned to the large "unknown" group. The research of the last few years, however, has disclosed that carriers of genes for recessive deafness may be identified from audiometric registration of certain peculiarities in the hearing function. In this connection it is of interest to note that the same types of peculiarties have been established in cases of verified sex-chromosome anomalies. This is an important advance not only as regards diagnostic work but also in the research into the genetics of deafness. On the basis of these research results it has been possible to demonstrate that the hearing loss in a child exposed to rubella during the first trimester of foetal life may well be the result of an interaction of endogenous and exogenous factors.

This paper surveys several studies concerning the aetiology of deafness, the titles of which and the names of collaborators are to be found in the reference list.

REFERENCES

Anderson, H. and Wedenberg, E. (1968). Audiometric identification of normal hearing carriers of genes for deafness. *Acta Otolaryng. Stockh.*, **65**, 535.

Anderson, H. and Wedenberg, E. (1970). Genetic aspects of hearing impairments in children. *Acta Otolaryng. Stockh.*, **69**, 77.

Anderson, H., Filipsson, R., Fluur, E., Koch, B., Lindsten, J. and Wedenberg, E. (1969). Hearing impairment in Turner's syndrome. *Acta Otolaryng. Stockh.*, Suppl. 247.

Anderson, H., Barr, B. and Wedenberg, E. (1970). Genetic disposition—a pre-requisite for maternal rubella deafness. *Arch. Otolaryng. Stockh.*, **91**, 141.

Anderson, H., Lindsten, J. and Wedenberg, E. (1971). Hearing defects in males with sex chromosome anomalies. *Acta Otolaryng. Stockh.*, **72**, 55.

Barr, B. and Lundström, R. (1961). Deafness following maternal rubella. *Acta Otolaryng. Stockh.*, **53**, 413.

Barr, B. and Wedenberg, E. (1964). Prognosis of perceptive hearing loss in children with respect to genesis and use of hearing aid. *Acta Otolaryng. Stockh.*, **59**, 462.

The Hearing Threshold—
Is it Measurable?

W. TEMPEST, R. M. BARR-HAMILTON
and M. E. BRYAN

Department of Electrical Engineering, University of Salford, England

At present, the most basic and widely used measure of the performance of the hearing process is the measurement of the air-conduction threshold, usually for pure tones. This concentration on the threshold would seem to be entirely justifiable, since it provides such an excellent screening test for hearing disorder. A normal threshold means in all but a very few cases, such as some instances of central deafness, normal hearing.

Although much use is made of threshold measurements it is perhaps not always realized how inaccurate are the conventional procedures. For instance at 1,000 Hz a change of the order of 10 dB must occur in repeated determinations before the change becomes significant in the statistical sense. At higher frequencies the change is in the region of 20 dB (Bryan and Tempest, 1967). Furthermore, the nature of the features of the hearing system which control the lower limit of sensitivity which we call the threshold is very little understood. This in turn implies that in measuring the threshold it is difficult to know whether the best possible techniques are being applied to the problem. The threshold is usually determined by a free choice procedure; in other words, a procedure in which the observer has to decide what criterion he is going to adopt in deciding when the signal has disappeared and when it appears again, the mean of the two signal levels at which these decisions are taken being regarded as the threshold. It is not surprising that the criterion adapted is open to many influences; for instance in this laboratory (Jacqueline A. Marsh, unpublished data) and at the National Physical Laboratory (Delaney, 1970) it has been found that the threshold of a naïve subject improves with practice. Delaney found "inexperienced subjects showed additional improvements due to familiarization varying from 1 to 9 dB". At Salford we have consistently found that experienced subjects in both MAF (minimum audible field) threshold measurements

31

(Hempstock *et al.*, 1966) and in MAP (minimum audible pressure) threshold measurements (Barr-Hamilton *et al.*, to be published) have about half the intra-subject variance of naïve subjects.

The word "threshold" itself is an unfortunate choice, since it suggests in everyday language a well-defined transition point between two regions, inaudibility and audibility, whilst it can be easily demonstrated experimentally that there is a region of uncertainty between the two.

In order to obtain a working hypothesis about the nature of the "threshold" without having any exact ideas about the precise physiology involved, it is necessary to proceed on a basis of such knowledge of the ear as can be gained from its measured performance, together with the physicist's knowledge of the general properties of matter, and where appropriate, by analogy with man-made systems such as microphones.

Considering first the microphone, the limiting sensitivity is provided by the noise generated at the microphone terminals in the absence of any acoustic input. This electrical noise output can be equated to an acoustic noise input to the microphone and it can generally be said that the microphone cannot be used to measure acoustic signals below this equivalent noise level, since such signals would produce an electrical output which would be lost in the microphone noise. Taking as a practical example a moving coil microphone, it is possible to regard the noise of the microphone as arising from the summing of three separate components, the electrical resistance of the coil, the mechanical resistance of the diaphragm suspension system, and the acoustic impedance (including a resistive term) of the air. In physical terms the noise sources all arise from the natural random motion of particles in the components concerned, electrons in the coil, molecules in the air and in the suspension. These basic noise sources which exist, in one form or another, in all forms of microphone, are fundamental, and can only be minimized by good design, never eliminated.

The ear is not a microphone, and does not work in the same way, but it is composed of atoms and molecules from the same universe and, so far as we know these atoms obey the same rules of behaviour everywhere, therefore the ear will have its own sources of noise, plus some extra ones due to its situation in a living animal. Figure 1 shows the possible location of (some of) the noise sources in the ear, in this case four are shown, air molecule noise, eardrum and middle ear mechanical resistance noise, blood-flow noise and neural noise.

At this stage two questions arise, first, have we any real evidence of the existence of these noise sources in the ear, and second, if they exist, what do they do to the ear's performance? The evidence for molecular noise in the air is both experimental and theoretical. Very minute dust particles in the air under a microscope move with the "Brownian"

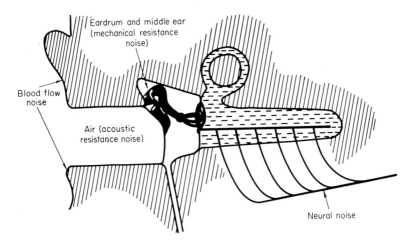

FIG. 1. Possible noise sources in the ear.

motion, due to collisions with air molecules, while Sivian and White (1933) calculated that the noise at the eardrum due to this effect was just below the threshold of audibility in the most sensitive part of the ear's range. The mechanical noise from the ear's physical structure can also be calculated, somewhat approximately, and again the answer is that the internal noise from the drum is just below the threshold of audibility. The actual noise level generated in an ear type cup by the ear (mainly by the blood flow) has been measured directly by Shaw and Piercy (1962) and by Anderson and Whittle (1971) and found to correspond fairly closely to the hearing threshold. It is difficult to say anything about neural noise, except that we know that nerve cells can fire randomly in the absence of a stimulus, and this could presumably be considered a form of noise.

If we accept the hypothesis that the ear has this noise, then we must consider whether it has any significant effect on its performance. The effect is to define the most sensitive threshold that the ear could have, if nature chose to make it so. In fact the measurements and calculations already mentioned show that this is probably the case, and that the ear, like the eye, is about as sensitive as nature will permit.

Having thus arrived at the premise that the ear at threshold may behave like a system limited in its sensitivity by internal noise, then the next problem is to test this by direct experiment. This is possible, by the application of the methods of statistical detection theory, which has been developed in connection with the ear's ability to distinguish signals from noise at relatively high intensities. The original (high intensity) supra-threshold work showed that if a listener is presented with a large number of signal presentations, against the background of noise at different levels in relation to the noise, then the proportion of the signals he will detect depends on the level, rising from zero when the signal is well below the noise, to 100 per cent when the signal is well above the noise. The actual transition from 0 to 100 per cent is not at all sudden, and occupies about 10 dB for a normal ear.

At the absolute threshold of hearing, i.e. with no external noise present—the transition from chance detection to 100 per cent detection is likewise about 10 dB wide and the ear behaves as if its threshold were determined by some form of noise (Barr-Hamilton et al., 1968; Eijkman and Vendrik, 1963).

Our experiment made use of the two interval forced-choice (2IFC) technique. The procedure has already been described in detail (Barr-Hamilton et al., 1968). In brief, two time intervals are indicated to the subject by lights: a signal is presented in one or the other of the intervals: then the subject must decide which interval he thinks most likely to have contained the signal.

The particular advantage of this technique is that it should eliminate the psychological factor which is present in conventional procedures, i.e. what criterion does the subject choose when deciding whether or not he heard a signal in a particular interval of time? Will he adopt a strict criterion, saying "I heard a signal" only when he was very sure a signal was present, or the opposite, a lax criterion? In the 2IFC procedure, the subject does not have to make a judgement of this type, as he is simply making a comparison of two intervals.

This should lead to a more precise measure of the threshold. Stephens (1969) has found that with two groups of subjects a forced choice procedure gave smaller intra-subject variance (the difference being significant at the 5 per cent level in four out of eight cases) than a standard free-choice procedure. Barr-Hamilton et al. (1969) compared the 2IFC technique with the Békésy method of audiometry, they found that the 2IFC procedure gave more sensitive thresholds, with no difference between the naïve and practiced subjects; the Békésy method showed an improvement in threshold sensitivity with practice.

In the present work the 2IFC procedure has been used as means of evaluating the threshold of hearing to give a criterion-free measure of sensitivity.

The method used estimated several points on the psychometric function, and it was therefore possible to use the results to give also a measure of the width of the psychometric function. Thus, in addition to being a threshold test, it lends itself to use as (yet another) test for cochlear lesion—one that is monaural, and can be used in cases of severe hearing loss (since it is not a supra-threshold test).

The measure of psychometric function width has been tentatively called the differential detectability index (DIDI). (Barr-Hamilton *et al.*, 1971.) The index was able to separate out the cases of cochlear lesion with a reliability of about 80 per cent. Figure 2 shows typical psycho-

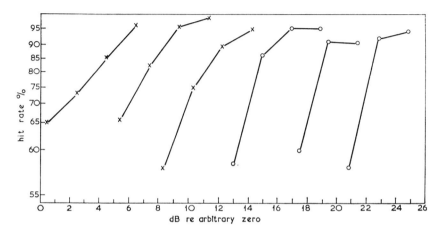

FIG. 2. Psychometric functions for some typical ears obtained using the 2IFC procedure: ——X—— normal ears; ——O—— cochlear-impaired ears.

metric functions obtained in our pilot study for some normal and coch-lear-impaired ears; the slope of the function tends to be greater in the latter cases, particularly in the narrow region closest to threshold. This result might suggest that the limiting factor which determines the threshold sensitivity is of a different nature in an ear with a cochlear lesion.

The 2IFC technique is at present being developed along the lines of a threshold-seeking device in which the signal level presented on each trial depends on the subject's responses on previous trials. The technique has a superficial similarity to the Békésy procedure, as the signal level will change from trial to trial, normally oscillating between a level slightly above threshold and a level slightly below. The range of the variation in the level is about 3 to 5 dB.

In a threshold-seeking system many possible decision rules regarding when to increase or decrease the signal level, and many rules concerning step size, may be formulated (e.g. see Wetherill and Levitt, 1965; Taylor and Creelman, 1967). In our first experiment using the apparatus, rules for changing the signal level were as shown in Table I. After each sequence, which contained up to four trials, a decision was made, the level was changed, and a new sequence was started. Under these

D

TABLE I

Decision Rules for Changing Signal Level

Response sequence	Decision
$+ + + +$	Decrease signal level by one step
$+ + + -$	Keep signal level constant
$+ + -$ or ⎫ $+ -$　or ⎬ $-$　　or ⎭	Increase signal level by one step

$+$ Correct response
$-$ False response

rules, the target level is the one at which the subject's hit rate is 82 per cent.

Like the decision rule, the step size is a variable that needs to be optimized, and depends on what the experimenter requires: if speed is required at the expense of some precision, a large step size is used; if precision is of prime importance and a longer test is acceptable, a smaller step size is used.

In a typical run illustrated in Fig. 3 the step size used was 1 dB. It is convenient to start the run some way above threshold, as this lets the subject familiarize himself with the procedure before the task becomes more difficult. Initially the signal level was reduced in steps of 5 dB using a manual attenuator; when the subject's responses indicated that

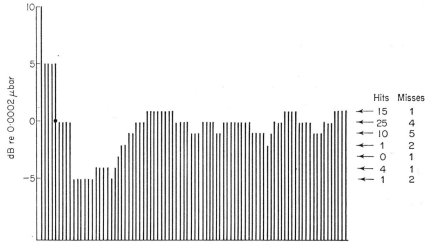

Fɪɢ. 3. A typical trace, of six min duration, obtained using the 2IFC threshold-seeking audiometer. The table at the right of the trace shows the number of "hits" and "misses" at each signal level.

the level was in the threshold region (i.e. after the first miss) the auto-matic system was put into operation.

It is evident from this example that the signal level can stabilize after quite a short time. The duration of this entire run was about 6 min, and it contained 86 trials, but clearly the test could have been concluded after about 4 min with only a small loss of accuracy. Also, the initial adjustment to the threshold region could be made more rapid. The threshold may be defined as the level at which the greatest number of trials was used: in this example 0 dB.

Another way of presenting the results is on a graph of hit rate against SPL as shown in Fig. 4. The data points are shown, together with an estimate of the standard deviation of each, and the psychometric func-tion was fitted by eye.

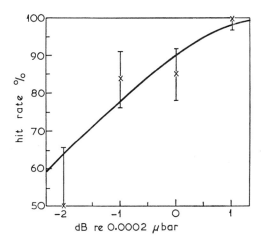

FIG. 4. A psychometric function drawn to data obtained in a run of the 2IFC threshold-seeking audiometer. An estimate of the standard deviation of each point is shown.

The technique is likely to be of particular value in the precise deter-mination of threshold, where there is need for a method that is indepen-dent of the criterion or skill of the observer. Although the technique and the instrumentation have been advanced to a stage where the 2IFC test can be given to a naïve listener, who can easily learn and complete the test in a few minutes, it has a disadvantage in being a little more difficult to learn than some tests, and the subject needs careful instruc-tion and sometimes a short practice. Hence its main use at this stage would be in laboratory work to measure small changes in acuity. Possibly a more sophisticated apparatus suitable for clinical use may be evolved from it.

REFERENCES

Anderson, C. M. B. and Whittle, L. S. (1971). Physiological noise and the missin 6 dB. *Acustica*, **24**, 261–272.

Barr-Hamilton, R. M., Bryan, M. E. and Tempest, W. (1968). The application of signal detection theory to the quiet threshold of hearing, *Sound*, **4**, 92–98.

Barr-Hamilton, R. M., Bryan, M. E. and Tempest, W. (1969). Applications of signal detection theory to audiometry, *Int. Audiol.*, **8**, 138–146.

Barr-Hamilton, R. M., Tempest, W. and Bryan, M. E. (1971). The differential detectability index: a new monaural test for the locus of hearing disorders? *Sound*, **5**, 2–6.

Bryan, M. E. and Tempest, W. (1967). Precision audiometry, *Acta oto-laryngologica*, **64**, 205–212.

Delaney, M. E. (1970). On the stability of auditory threshold, *NPL Aero Report Ac*, **44**.

Eijkman, E. and Vendrik, A. J. H. (1963). Detection theory applied to the absolute sensitivity of sensory systems. *Biophys. J.*, **3**, 65–68.

Hempstock, T. I., Bryan, M. E. and Webster, J. B. C. (1966). Free-field threshold variance, *J. Sound Vib.*, **4**, 33–44.

Sataloff, J. (1966). "Hearing Loss". Lippincott, Co., Philadelphia.

Shaw, E. A. G. and Piercy, J. E. (1962). "Audiometry and Physiological Noise". Paper H46 IVth ICA Copenhagen.

Sivian, L. J. and White, S. D. (1933). *J. acoust. Soc. Am.*, **4**, 288–321.

Stephens, S. D. G. (1969). Auditory threshold variance, signal detection theory and personality, *Int. Audiol.*, **8**, 131–137.

Taylor, M. M. and Creelman, C. D. (1967). PEST: efficient estimates of probability functions, *J. acoust. Soc. Am.* **41**,, 782–787.

Wetherill, C. B. and Levitt, H. (1965). Sequential estimation of points on a psychometric function, *Brit. J. Math. Statistical. Psychol.*, **18**, 1–10.

Practical Aspects of Ascertainment of Young Children with Hearing Defects

M. DUNN and E. S. McGREGOR

School Health Service, Glasgow, Scotland, and
Education Department, Glasgow, Scotland

INTRODUCTION

Glasgow is the largest city in Scotland with a population of about 1,000,000. The child population under five years is about 80,000 with a birth rate of about 20,000 per year.

Our discussion is confined to five cases, all under five years, presenting diagnostic assessment, and placement problems, and we will indicate our solutions based on our resources and the philosophy of our area as regards education.*

These children have been referred to the Balvicar Centre in whcih Elizabeth McGregor is the Educational Audiologist, and I am the Local Authority Medical Officer—my function is Specialist Medical Officer, Hearing, with regard to School Health Service in Glasgow and assessment and ascertainment of any under 5-year-old who comes to our notice, under the Education (Scotland) Act 1969.

The Balvicar Centre was opened in 1964—it had a grant from the Carnegie U.K. Trust. It aims at providing treatment and support for all forms of medical, social and emotional defects in children in the under-5 age group. In this Centre, Elizabeth McGregor is housed in a purpose-built Audiology Unit. Investigation in her department can be linked up through myself to the medical team carrying out developmental paediatrics in the same Centre and thus much can be contained in this one area, making for ease of availability of assessment for children and parents and avoiding fragmentation of services and communications. It also keeps the investigation and follow-up in the community which is a necessity in this work.

Our scheme of action is outlined in "Ascertainment of Children with Hearing Defects, Scottish Education Department, 1967".

* The five cases detailed are not included in this published record.

In this respect we have our inner, first line team:

1. Otologist
2. Medical Officer of Local Authority
3. Educational Audiologist
4. Educational Psychologist

Attached by various linkages are:

Paediatrician	Health Visitor
Neurologist	Social Worker
Psychiatrist	Speech Therapist

Glasgow, with its million population, is more fortunate than many other Scottish areas in its screening facilities and provision for the education of hearing impaired children. We do, however, still have many problems and are conscious of these. I shall outline some of these briefly.

There is the very thorny problem of placement of language disordered children with apparently normal or near normal peripheral hearing. In Glasgow staff and accommodation are at a premium. Therefore the availability of personnel for research into the most valid methods of guidance for these specific difficulties is necessarily limited.

Also a problem is that of differential diagnosis when language difficulties cloud the issue—we don't speak Urdu or Punjabi.

The provision of a "partially hearing" unit in an ordinary school must be envisaged in the near future and serious consideration given to the placement problems of academically retarded, hearing impaired children who are unable to cope with oral methods of education.

The assessment and guidance of children in remote areas is also a problem. Glasgow has accepted the responsibility of this service for Argyll and the Western Islands. A start has been made towards the provision of a postal programme.

Financial help for travelling for diagnostic assessment is available—the question of whether this is widely enough known or used is equivocal. When no reason is forthcoming for continuous non-attendance, it is difficult to find out if it is purely lack of finance—or perhaps lack of parental interest.

Of immediate concern to the Unit is the dissemination of information and publicity to encourage not only Local Authorities but also G.P.s, E.N.T. Consultants, Paediatricians, Speech Therapists, etc., to make early and comprehensive use of the facilities available. Perhaps then we shall no longer find, as happens on occasion, a 4-year-old not communicating adequately, due to a hearing impairment!

We have been discussing aspects of ascertainment and guidance at the "grass roots" level; but this is where we work, in the field, with children who have communication difficulty.

Threshold of Hearing in Children— Some Difficulties

T. S. RUSSELL

The Victoria Infirmary, Glasgow, Scotland

I would like to describe some of the problems that arose during the survey that we recently completed, and published, in the hope that you might find some of our experiences helpful, and an awful warning.

We found that the problems sorted themselves into four main groups: general design, materials required, specific audiometric techniques and their recording, and compilation and presentation of the results. I will deal with each in turn.

We were interested in developing standards for the thresholds of hearing by air conduction in children. Now, in deriving population standards, it is logically desirable to measure every individual but this is rarely, if ever, possible, and it therefore becomes necessary to adopt some policy which will produce a reliable sample. Some sampling procedures can be controlled by statistical methods, but we thought it unlikely that we could deal with large enough numbers to develop statistically reliable figures for all ages. Since the previous standard, young adult surveys used 18–25 years as their age limits, we decided, because of the ages of school populations, to sample at half-decade intervals, i.e. at 5, 10, 15, years of age. This required modification because compulsory education terminates at the age of 15 years, so that we had to accept the 14th year as the best compromise. It is important to remember that we could have obtained adequate numbers of children aged 15 years, but these would have been selected by the loss of the poorer children who generally leave school soon after their 15th birthday.

We were agreed that, with the estimated numbers we would require, there was no possibility of finding sufficient children in one school, nor any hope of transporting the children to a central testing area, and we would thus require mobility of our testing equipment. This assumption was well founded, especially with the 5 year olds who are mostly in smaller schools, and we sometimes visited schools for as few as five completed results, especially during the winter when children might be absent, or have infected ears. As a matter of interest, we visited upwards of 40 schools, ranging from the smallest primary to huge comprehensive with up to 300 children in one age group.

In conformity with the previous standard studies, we decided to use only otologically normal children. To satisfy this criterion, each child was examined, and rejected if either ear showed wax concealing more than one third of the tympanic membrane, foreign bodies, otitis externa, acute otitis media, secretory otitis media—active or inactive, or chronic suppurative otitis media.

It will be clear that these obvious otological abnormalities only excluded from the survey most of the causes of conductive deafness, and that we would still be committed to measuring and including children with some types of conductive deafness, and any type of perceptive deafness. We hoped that by rigidly categorizing our rejections, it would be possible to ensure comparability between surveys, but this comparability suffered sadly in other ways.

The materials needed were two only, silence and a source of sound. In our world the former is more expensive by far, the more so as it had to be transportable. With much help, and welcome advice from Dr Taylor, we designed a caravan consisting of a weighted outer shell, surrounding a standard double acoustic booth. The mobility was assured by a steerable front axle to which the towing eye was attached. The transport, and maintenance of this vehicle was the largest recurrent difficulty that we encountered. The caravan weighs a little more than three tons, and for safety requires a towing vehicle of about the same weight. It could be towed, as in fact it was, by an ex-army Austin weighing a little less than a ton. At other times we had the use of the Cleansing Department collecting vehicle, a South of Scotland Electricity Board lorry, and on two occasions it travelled on a low loader. On one of these visits the low loader nudged a brick-built gate post which collapsed at once, and was not revived for about two years. We never had any reliable, or constant source of transport, and I would therefore advise for the future that any van be self-propelled, or that care be taken at an early stage in the trailer design to ensure that a suitable towing vehicle will be available. When divorced from any source of mechanical power the mobility of the van was more theoretical than practical, except on a sloping playground, where special care had to be taken to make sure that none of the experimentally minded children could ease off the parking brake. There was no possible way of preventing the same children from unscrewing the lights on the outside of the van, or decorating it with assorted inscriptions, some painted, some incised, and so the van became lightless and increasingly decorated as the survey proceeded. We were very grateful to the children of one primary school who did not spread the news that the valve caps could be unscrewed, and the tyres let down with a matchstick. These high pressure tyres cannot be inflated with a foot pump, and before we discovered how to inflate them with compressed air cylinders the wheels had to be removed, one at a time, after jacking up the van, and transported to the nearest garage for inflation. I should say that we were always careful to immobilize the outer door padlock before settling to work inside, and we never had to use the escape panel and hatchet provided.

For its prime purpose this trailer was very suitable, and was acoustically satisfactory. No ventilation was fitted to either the inner booth, or the outer shell, and we never had any need of it. With two people inside it never became unpleasantly hot, and, in fact, some extra heating was required on cold winter days. The doors of the van and the booth gave some little trouble, and I would say that this is the most difficult part of any silent room, and the one where most reward could come from experimentation.

By contrast the sound sources were easy. Early surveys had to develop their own equipment, we had only to procure reliable audiometers. We bought a pair of Peters basic diagnostic audiometers which we calibrated regularly, and checked for output each morning. They were modified for our purpose in two ways: first to read down to -20 dB and second by removal of the click stops on the attenuater control. This had to be done after we discovered that their presence was biasing the 2 dB interval readings very heavily in favour of the 10 dB points.

The test procedure and its recording had only two obvious difficulties. It is always preferable to have the subject isolated in a booth, but we felt that 5-year-old children would not tolerate this situation, and we therefore arranged that the audiometrician would be in the booth with the child. Although this might produce some masking noise, well-fitting ear caps should control this adequately. The second difficulty here is the problem of rejection of results by the audiometrician, as being non-standard. The simplest solution for this is the use of an automatic recording audiometer, but no satisfactory instrument is available. We circumvented this by laying down a rigid procedure for the examination, with all results recorded. I may outline the procedure by saying that after a trial presentation at 1,000 cps, each frequency was examined separately in a predetermined order. The sequence was to present a suprathreshold tone, lower the intensity until no tone was perceptible, then raise again for a perceptible tone. The threshold crossing was repeated twice more in each direction. This procedure was intended to correspond reasonably well with the method of an automatic audiometer, but to be swifter and as accurate. It also confoms with normal audiometric practice, only excepting the assessment of the "threshold level" by the audiometrician.

I am sorry to say that in spite of all our care with the selection and calibration of equipment, it was necessary to standardize the survey by running a short series on young adults. This resulted from the fact that, in spite of all the calibration technique presently available, nothing can completely compensate for different equipment. Previous surveys had used S.T.C. earphones, and we were using telephonics. The error would not be expected to be large, but it does exist, and could not be corrected by any means that we could devise. This is certainly a major defect in present equipment, and only emphasizes that some alternative is needed to present earphone listening techniques, with their constant vulnerability to minor damage.

The compilation and presentation of results was eased, in some ways, by the availability of a computer, but the ease with which it operated meant that we were tempted to ask for more details extracted from the raw data than we could well use. In the end our final presentation included only some of the simplest histograms of threshold against number of observations, and multiple graphs of frequency against threshold levels. The numerical presentation runs to four closely printed pages which are completely indigestible, therefore Fig. 1 shows the frequency along the receding axis, against the amplitude on the horizontal axis.

The area in which we expected most difficulty—the handling and

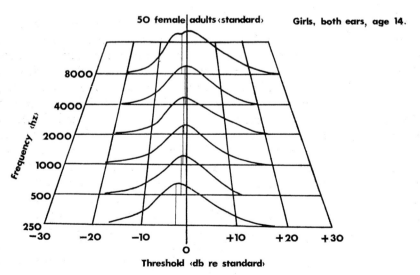

FIG. 1. Histogram showing comparison of thresholds between 50 female adults and girls aged 14 years.

testing of large numbers of children—proved to be almost trouble free, as did the direct recording of a completely standardized type of threshold testing suitable for transference to a computer input.

Our results have good internal consistency, and agree well with previous surveys, demonstrating a threshold for 9 year olds (see Fig. 2)

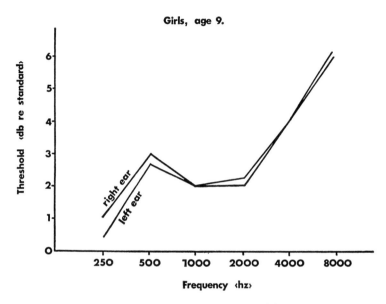

FIG. 2. Hearing thresholds of girls aged 9 years.

comparable to that of adults, with the 5 year olds being poorer, and the 14 year olds better. There is a small group of children at all ages whose hearing threshold is greatly better than the standard, and the histograms, which otherwise have a normal bell-shaped distribution pattern, almost all show a small bump at the −20 dB level. It seems possible that there is something to be learned from further investigation of this group of children.

Neuro-Physiological Tests in Audiometry

H. A. BEAGLEY

The Institute of Laryngology and Otology,
England

Et personne ne met du vin nouveau dans de veilles outres; sinon, le vin fera éclater les outres, et le vin est perdu ainsi que les outres. Mais à vin nouveau outres neuves!

Saint Marc

One is warned of the danger of putting new wine into old wineskins—and the converse too, for that matter. But we may rest assured on this point for, while neurophysiological tests of hearing are sufficiently fresh to be regarded as new wine, the First Conference of the British Society of Audiology is certainly no "old" wineskin.

Neurophysiological tests of hearing at present in use, or under active investigation and development, include the central phenomena such as the early cortical potential, the slow cortical potential (the well-known auditory evoked response) and the slow d.c. potentials. From the periphery we can record the auditory nerve action potential and the cochlear microphonic. As all of these bio-electric potentials are most easily demonstrated by some form of electronic averaging, and the general term "electric response audiometry" is considered wide enough to include them all. While most of these bio-electric potenials are of interest mainly in the field of research, two are sufficiently developed to be of practical use in the field of clinical audiometry. These are:

1. The auditory evoked cortical response, generally called "evoked response audiometry", which will be discussed mainly in this paper, and:
2. The VIII nerve action potential (electro-cochleogram) which will be discussed in the following paper.

It will be seen immediately that the first records a central cortical response to an acoustic stimulus, while the second is entirely peripheral

47

in origin, and this physiological difference has considerable potential advantages in the context of clinical investigation.

In a minority of difficult clinical cases, it is not possible to get reliable subjective estimates of the patients' hearing threshold by means of conventional audiometry and in such cases recourse may be made to evoked response audiometry. The patient's judgement is not required, as in conventional audiometry, because the tester decides whether or not there is a response, and the method is sometimes called "objective". This is true as far as the subject is concerned, but the tester's decision is, of course, still subjective. However, it is often better to remove the onus of judgement from an unreliable or unco-operative subject. But in the majority of cases there is no reason to prefer the so-called objective test to the conventional pure tone audiogram.

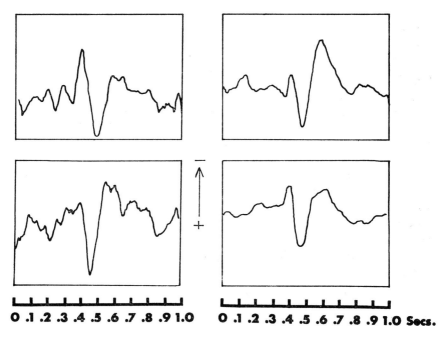

0 .1 .2 .3 .4 .5 .6 .7 .8 .9 1.0   0 .1 .2 .3 .4 .5 .6 .7 .8 .9 1.0 Secs.

FIG. 1. This illustration shows commonly occurring patterns of the auditory evoked response. In each case, the response is 70 dB above threshold and the stimulus used is at 0·3 sec. Note the variable second negative wave (N_2). This is often seen in young adults and frequently predominate in children. (Reprinted from *J. Laryng.*)

The auditory evoked cortical potential can be produced by any audible sound with a fairly abrupt onset. Short pulses of pure tones are generally used, with a rise-decay time of 10–30 millisec. As the evoked response is small with respect to the on-going EEG rhythms, it is necessary to summate the response to a series of stimuli, say 30 to 100, using an electronic averager—usually a small digital computer—which summates the identical evoked responses selectively so that they can be readily identified, thereby providing a physiological indicator. As this can be done at various frequencies and intensities, it forms the basis of a method of audiometry.

Contrary to what was formerly thought, the auditory evoked response is not a non-specific phenomenon originating in the association areas of the brain, but as Vaughan's (1968) mapping experiments have shown, it is actually a specific response from the primary auditory area in the temporal lobe and is best recorded between an electrode on the vertex and another below the base of the skull, usually in the mastoid region. This is the electrode placement most frequently used in clinical hearing testing by this method. The time course of the response is slow, lasting from 50 millisec. from the onset of the stimulus to 2–300 millisec. as shown in Fig. 2. The P_1–N_1–P_2 nomenclature as used by Davis (1964), is used to denote the polarity of the response. Other characteristics of

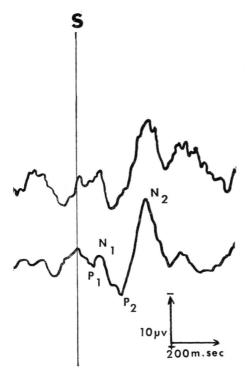

FIG. 2. This shows the trace of an aphasic child (*below*) and a non-aphasic child (*above*) showing that the responses are essentially similar. (Reprinted from *Sound*.)

the response are that there is a parallel relation between the response amplitude and the intensity of the sound stimuli, except at very high intensities, where the amplitude of the evoked response tends to level off. The amplitude of the response is also closely related to the interval between the sound stimuli, longer interstimulus intervals producing larger amplitudes. This is attributed to greater cortical recovery (Davis *et al.*, 1966). Frequency is not an important variable except above 4 kHz, when less amplitude growth is seen.

As the purpose of the test is to use the cortical evoked response as a physiological indicator, a compromise must be struck so as to get the maximum response amplitude within a reasonable time. Therefore, a series of about 50 stimuli is frequently used, with an interstimulus interval of 1–2 sec. At each frequency tested, a suprathreshold recording of the response is made at 50–60 dB above threshold. This is repeated at successively lower levels of intensity until the evoked response can no longer be positively identified. Usually this is about 5–10 dB above the subject threshold, or even a little less (Beagley and Kellog, 1969). In this way the evoked response threshold is established, and it must be stressed that this always is higher than the subjective threshold, due to the remaining background noise—i.e. the evoked response threshold is always a little less sensitive than the subjective threshold in adults, and more so in the case of young children.

In adults it is only very rarely that one is unable to establish the patient's threshold by evoked response testing, even in those individuals who produce a very small cortical response. But central abnormalities can sometimes cause difficulties. Epileptiform discharges may effectively mask the response, while cerebral thrombosis causing bilateral lesions of the temporal lobes with deafness and nominal aphasia similarly prevented the registration of the evoked response in one particular case. Other lesions, however, have failed to suppress the response, e.g. in the case of an adult whose skull fracture has been repaired by a large metallic plate. In this case there was no difficulty in recording the evoked response and establishing the auditory threshold by this means (Beagley, 1971) (Fig. 3.).

Children can also be tested by this method, and indeed young children who may be otherwise untestable are the most important potential group of patients for whom evoked response testing is appropriate. Except that the EEG background tends to be large and the evoked response a little more variable, there is very little difficulty in testing school-age children, given at least passive co-operation. In general, with this age group it is possible to establish the evoked response threshold with about 10 dB of the subjective threshold.

A very important group of school-age children who may be investi-

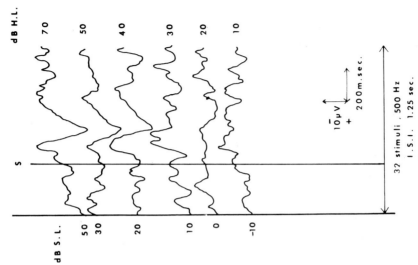

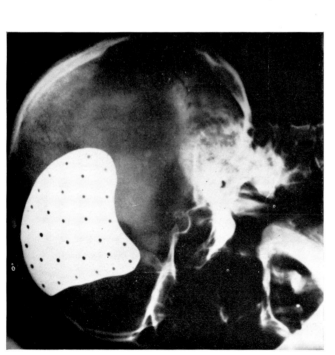

F IG . 3. A series of quite typical evoked responses from an adult who had suffered a severe head injury necessitating the insertion of a large metal plate. This did not prevent his hearing being assessed by this method.

E

gated by this technique are those suspected of having a receptive aphasia. Although true receptive aphasia is a rare condition, frequently the result of an acute febrile episode such as encephalitis, but occasionally having no antecedent history and therefore presumed to be developmental in origin, nevertheless the definitive diagnosis can present some problems. This is because, sometimes, a child who is severely deaf cannot be adequately distinguished from a normally hearing child with aphasia. By definition, the aphasic's speech problem is not related to hearing loss and most have quite normal hearing. Evoked response testing has been effective in separating these children from straightforward cases of deafness. In fact, the auditory evoked response presents no particular features which are different from the evoked responses of non-aphasic children (Beagley, 1970), contrary to what has been claimed by some investigators, as shown in Fig. 2. Pre-school children and young infants are an important group as a proportion will resist

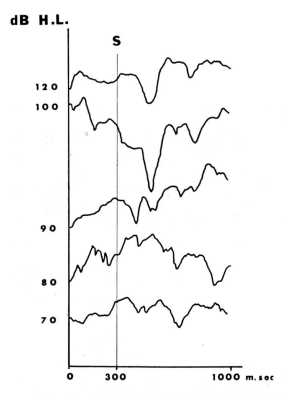

Fɪɢ. 4. D.J. 4½ years. This series of traces (at 500Hz) indicates that this child's threshold is in the region of 80dB H.L. The response was traced down to 90dB, but the trace at 80dB was indeterminate and was considered to correspond with her actual hearing threshold.

efforts to assess them by the usual subjective methods. Evoked response testing can be carried out in these children either awake, or in natural sleep, or if necessary, under sedation. Ideally, the child is best tested awake, and Fig. 4 shows the response from one of a pair of twins who developed considerable hearing loss by the age of 4 years, despite the early acquisition of speech. Evoked response testing confirmed that each child had developed a severe hearing loss of 80 dB average in the better ear and one twin actually had a virtually dead ear on one side; the pathology was almost certainly rubella embryopathy and the evoked response testing confirmed a finding which would otherwise have been difficult to accept on clinical grounds. In the 2 to 4 year age group, the sensitivity gap between the evoked response threshold and the mean adult threshold widens to about 20 dB and in the neonatal period it may be as much as 40 dB.

If the child to be tested is turbulent or hyperactive, it may be impossible to apply the electrodes and conduct the test, or the results may be compromised by a profusion of movement artefacts due to potentials from the neck muscles contaminating the records. Sedation is therefore required and workers in various countries are looking into this problem.

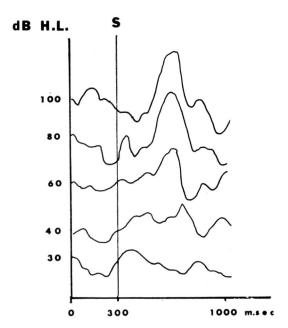

Fig. 5. Female 3½ years, Phenergan sedation, 1k H₂ tone. This series of traces shows how the threshold of hearing can be established in young children. As this child was too nervous to test awake, she was sedated with intramuscular Phenergan and was tested during sleep. Her threshold, at this frequency, was estimated to be between 30 and 40 dB.

Non-barbiturate sedation is preferred by most, but not all, investigators, and Largactil, Chloralhydrate, Valium, Vallergan and Phenergan have have all been used (Fig. 5). Consistently satisfactory results have been reported by the use of Phenergan intra-muscularly and this drug is now used routinely for evoked response testing. On the other hand, anaesthesia has not really proved to be satisfactory for evoked response testing.

The extraction of the cortical evoked response still poses some problems in some young children and infants, especially those with brain damage. No doubt more sophisticated methods of signal extraction will help to resolve this problem, but, alternatively, it may be avoided by using a different type of neuro-physiological measurement which is showing great promise clinically. This is recording of the VIII nerve action potential, the electro-cochleogram which has been perfected very largely by Aran, Portmann and Le Bert. This is purely a peripheral

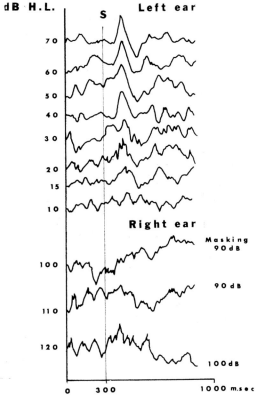

FIG. 6. This patient, an adult female, produced the above traces in the left ear, right ear, respectively, in response to a series of 1 kHz test tones. It indicates that her hearing level is between 10 and 15 dB in the left ear and between 100 and 110 dB in the right ear.

measurement and as each ear is tested separately and in isolation, masking is unnecessary. One disadvantage is that frequency information is restricted, but another great advantage is that the test can be carried out under general anaesthesia, which can be a decisive factor in the case of some hyperactive infants.

Thus it can be seen that at least two electrophysiological methods, evoked response testing and electro-cochleography, have reached the stage of clinical usefulness and others may well follow. It is also clear that these two used in conjunction would permit the diagnosis of central deafness to be either confirmed or refuted.

As far as evoked response testing is concerned, this has been established a little longer than electro-cochleography, and while some experience is required to get the best results, the following clinical situations lend themselves to elucidation by this method.

1. In the case of unreliable or unrepeatable pure tone audiograms which need confirmation.
2. The investigation of suspected non-organic hearing loss.
3. The identification of simulators, in the Services or in industry.
4. In the case of young children untestable by reason of mental retardation or hyperactivity.
5. In children suspected of receptive aphasia, to confirm the presence or absence of hearing.
6. In deaf-blind children who are almost impossible to test in any other way.

And finally it must be stressed that electric, or evoked, response audiometry is only required when conventional subjective methods are either inconclusive or impossible to apply. It is in no sense a substitute for conventional pure tone audiometry.

REFERENCES

Beagley, H. A. (1970). *Sound*, **4**, 62.
Beagley, H. A. *J. Laryng.* (In press.)
Beagley, H. A. and Kellogg, S. E. (1969). *Int. Audiol.*, **8**, 345.
Davis, H. (1964). *Acta Otolaryng. Stockh.*, Supp. **206**, 128.
Davis, H., Mast, T., Yoshie, N. and Zerlin, S. (1966). *EEG-Clin. Neurol.*, **21**, 105.
Portmann, M., Aran, J-M. and Le Bert, G. (1968). *Acta Otolaryng. Stockh.*, **65**, 105.
Vaughan, H. G. (1968). *N.A.S.A. Symposium S.P.*, **191**, 45.

Electro-Cochleography in Babies

J.-M. ARAN* and M. PORTMANN

*Laboratoire D'Audiologie Experimentale, Faculté de Médicine
de Bordeaux, Bordeaux, France*

We have found the method of electro-cochleographic recordings developed in our research laboratory, very useful, when applied to the clinic, particularly in children (Aran and Le Bert, 1968; Aran, 1971a).

By now, more than 100 children have been tested, their ages ranging from one month to 6 years, most of them being between 2 and 4 years old. Of course, the recordings, which require perforation of the tympanic membrane with a thin needle electrode, are performed under light general anaesthesia induced by Ketamin (Aran *et al.*, 1969). In such a way testing both ears is possible very rapidly and with the best reliability.

The electro-cochleographic tests give us precise information on the function of each peripheral receptor, not only with respect to the thresholds, to the clicks, and the different filtered clicks, but also concerning the dynamics of the ear and the quality of the coding in the auditory nerve. For instance, we find the different patterns observed in adults corresponding to different pathological conditions (Aran, 1971b): the recruiting, broad, abnormal responses corresponding to sensori-neural disorders respectively at the levels of the cochlea, eighth nerve and retro-cochlear area.

Some particular results concerning children can be pointed out (Aran, 1971c; Portmann and Aran, 1971). The normal response (which is fortunately observed quite often in children who do not react normally to sound) has a shorter latency at the threshold ($\simeq 4$ millisec.) than for adults (5–6 millisec.). The recruiting response, image of lesions mainly of the sensori and/or neural external structures of the Organ of Corti, and evidence of pronounced loudness recruitment, is occasionally observed. The dissociated response has never been observed up to now. This pattern seems to correspond in the adult to occupational deafness with hearing loss only on the high frequencies. An abnormal response is observed, as in the adult, in complex neurological syndromes which could imply a lesion both in the cochlear and retro-cochlear area. It is

* Chargé de Recherche, I.N.S.E.R.M.

often observed in kernicterus cases. Since we know that, in the adult, such an abnormal pattern, no matter what the threshold is, corresponds to very poor speech discrimination, we can infer that for the child there will be difficulty in auditory and speech training. This is more than could be expected from the auditory threshold which in some cases can be relatively good (around 30 dB).

Thus it appears that electro-cochleography is an invaluable technique for the care of young children and babies who appear to have hearing difficulties. The function of each of the two peripheral receptors can be clearly demarcated and measured, and from these measurements a precise therapeutic procedure can be safely proposed.

REFERENCES

Aran, J.-M. (1971a). L'Electro-Cochléogramme, I—Principe et Technique; II— Résultats. *Les Cahiers de la C.F.A.*, Paris.

Aran, J-M. (1971b). Clinical Measures of VIIIth nerve Function (presented at the International Symposium on Oto-Physiology, Ann-Arbor, Michigan, May 1971). *Adv. Otolaryngol.* (In press.)

Aran, J.-M. (1971c). The Electro-Cochleogram: recent results in children and in some pathological cases, *Arch. Klin. exp. Ohr. –, Nas, – u. Kehlk. Heilk.* **198**, 128–141.

Aran, J.-M. and Le Bert, G. (1968). Les réponses nervouses cochléaires chez l'homme—image du fonctionnement de l'oreille et nouveau test d'audiométrie objective, *Rev. Laryng. Bordeaux*, **89**, 361–378.

Aran, J.-M., Portmann, Cl., Delaunay, J., Pelerin, J. and Lenoir, J. (1969). L'Electro-Cochléogramme: Méthode et premiers résultats chez l'enfant, *Rev. Laryng. Bordeaux*, **90**, 615–634.

Portmann, M. and Aran, J.-M. (1971). Electro-Cochleographie sur le nourisson et le jeune enfant, *Acta Otolaryng. Stockh.*, **71**, 253–261.

The Use of Fast Correlators in Electro-Cochleography in Man

W. D. KEIDEL

Physiologisches Institut der Universitat,
Erlangen-Nurnberg, Erlangen, West Germany

There are several papers about efforts to record the so-called early responses and especially the compound action potential of the auditory nerve in man, for example those by Yoshie (1968); Aran *et al.* (1970) and others. The highest amplitudes can be recorded when using electrodes which penetrate the ear drum and which are situated somewhere near the round window of a human ear. On the other hand, it is tempting to try to find clear responses to special types of stimuli by means of either the averaging or the auto- and cross-correlation technique, including the use of electronic computers. Looking at the history of this technique, the work of Dr Salomon in Denmark should be mentioned, also the fact that the equipment necessary for the recording of electrical responses of the human ear in this manner is considerably large and cannot conveniently be used in hospitals, as would be desirable for the benefit of deaf children.

To overcome all those problems and to improve the technology in two respects, namely, first, a much smaller device and, second, a reliable and great enough amplitude of N_1 and N_2, we used a special type of electrodes situated on the hard palate in human subjects. For this procedure it is necessary to have a special polyester set-up with two silver plates sitting on both sides of the hard palate, thus enabling one to separate the responses from the left and right side as related to the left and right ear. A picture of these electrodes is shown in Fig. 1. Although it is relatively easy to prepare the device for holding the silver electrodes, we are now also trying to use electrodes held by vacuum, which eliminates the necessity of a special adaptation to the shape of the palate of any given individual.

As the next figure shows, by means of the normal averaging technique (special program developed by Dr Finkenzeller in our department; LINC 8) we could obtain clear N_1 and N_2 responses on a 10 millisec

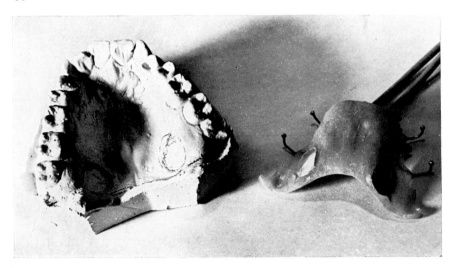

FIG. 1. Left: Mould of palate and upper teeth of the subject. Right: Palate plate for the electrode container with fastening clamps and with the silver electrodes. The positions of the electrodes on the palate can be recognized in the mould on the left side.

time scale. The stimuli are shown at the bottom of Fig. 2a. They do not show the electrical pattern, but the mechanical impulses delivered to an ear-phone after careful filtering. It is very important to have the clicks shaped as well as possible in order to obtain reliable and good results. Furthermore, having the stimuli delivered alternatingly, so that each even number of pulses within the train is a condensation click and each odd number is a rarefaction click, is very helpful in avoiding disturbance by electrical artifacts and microphonic potentials. With this technique nearly any electrical artifact and nearly any microphonic potential can easily be excluded. In the first series of experiments, a repetition rate of two per second was used and a few thousand single stimuli were necessary in order to obtain a good signal-to-noise ratio. The signal-to-noise ratio can be improved by increasing the number of stimuli. In our case, a compromise was observed somewhere around 5,000 stimuli. The intensities as well as the latencies are clearly related to the intensity of the stimuli delivered to the ear-phones on both ears. This can be seen better in Fig. 2b, which is the record of only condensation click responses, but to different intensities, so that the electrical artifact (E), the cochlear microphonics (CM), and the N_1 and N_2 responses can be clearly separated. It is very easy to separate those four types of electrical activities, namely, first, the electrical artifact (thick solid line), second, the cochlear microphonics (thin solid line), and third and fourth, the N_1 and N_2 responses to the clicks.

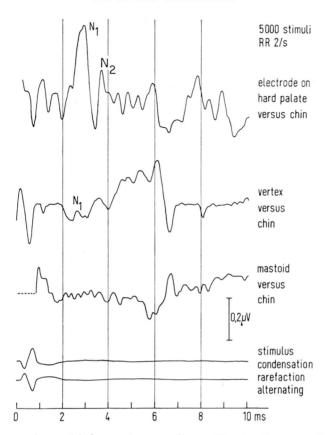

F ɪɢ. 2a. Averaged potentials from various recording positions by alternating stimulus form
(condensation and rarefaction).

Again, the first series of experiments, where condensation and rarefaction clicks were alternatingly delivered to the human subject's ear
(male subject; age 32 years), show that the size of a N_1 response recorded
with the palate electrode at an intensity of 70 dB above threshold is in
the order of only 0·2 microvolts, even after averaging. Although this is
only $\frac{1}{100}$ of the size of the evoked response recorded from vertex (about
20 μ volts), it is still about 10 to 20 times greater than when recorded
from any other place in the mouth, or at the ear lobe, or at the mastoid,
or at the vertex. So there is no doubt that by using this special electrode
the greatest amplitude of this response can be recorded. On the other
hand, in relation to the information processing within the auditory
channel up to the auditory cortex, quite a few other "early responses"
can be recorded, for instance one showing up somewhere between 6 and
10 millisec. after onset of the stimulus Figure 2a shows a comparison of

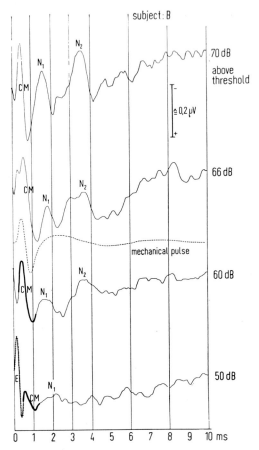

F IG. 2b. Averaged responses to condensation clicks of different intensities RR 4/s.

the size of this potential when one records simultaneously from the palate electrode (upper trace), from vertex (middle trace), and from mastoid (lower trace). Although the size for N_1 and N_2 is greatest at the palate, the size of the response with a latency of 6 to 8 millisec is biggest from the vertex electrode and is just detectable at the mastoid. On the other hand, all records from mastoid are certainly worse than those recorded from palate and vertex. In addition, there is a third "early response" which appears with a latency between 15 and 30 millisec after onset of stimulus. This response is shown in Fig. 3 as a function of intensity and clearly shows amplitude and latency shift with changing intensities.

   If we reconsider for a moment the results obtainable by using this special hard palate electrode, they can be divided into four events with

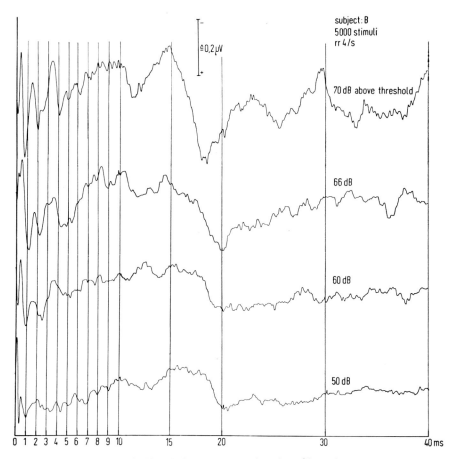

FIG. 3. Electrical response as a function of intensity.

latencies of 1, 2, 6 to 10, and 15 to 30 millisec; the two latter ones are probably the same as those described with other techniques by Dan Geisler, Nelson Kiang and Robert Goldstein, respectively. It is clear that by recording all those events simultaneously, with or without the microphonic potentials, by using either condensation clicks alone or condensation and rarefaction clicks alternatingly, the information available along the auditory pathway is considerably expanded in relation to techniques where just one of those components is a goal of the recording. We therefore believe that the use of this special electrode might be helpful in the future, even if just using the simple averaging technique and any type of a small computer like the LINC 8 or even the CAT, or a comparable small fixed-programmed computer, for clinical use.

In addition, if one looks at the potentials which can be obtained by recording from the vertex position of electrodes of the usual type, three more events can be looked at, namely, first, the well-known V-potential with medium latencies around 90 to 250 millisec and, second, when using long-lasting continuous tones or long-lasting trains of clicks with very high repetition rates, a dc-potential negative on vertex versus any other place for the indifferent electrode can be recorded, as we have shown in a series of papers published elsewhere (David *et al.*, 1969). As a third event of these medium and long latency type responses, the off-effect to the cessation of the long-lasting tone is usually interacting with the cut-off of the type of dc-potential, which is clearly different from Gray Walter's expectancy potential and from Kornhuber's motor potentials, described elsewhere. This is shown in Fig. 4, where a comparison of all seven events, the four early components and the three late responses, is simultaneously recorded by leading off from only two electrodes simultaneously, namely, the palate electrode and the vertex

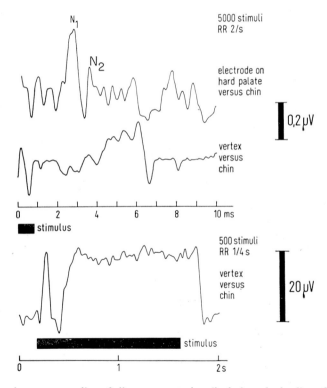

FIG. 4. Simultaneous recording of all seven events described above by leading off from only two electrodes simultaneously. A 10 millisec scale has been chosen for the early responses which allows particularly the N_1 and N_2 and the responses with latencies of 6 to 8 millisec to stand out.

electrode in the same subject. All seven of those responses, which are due to different levels within the auditory channnel, are of clinical importance and can lead to a separation and differential diagnosis in clinical cases because they allow one to separate and to define at which level, from periphery up to cortical level, they are originated. The technology available now and developed at our department during the past years suggests two types of records, namely, a time scale of 10 or of 40 millisec for the early responses, where the latter emphasizes the 15 to 30 millisec latency response, and a two-second time scale for the vertex potential. This latter type of recording is shown in Fig. 5. One can clearly see by

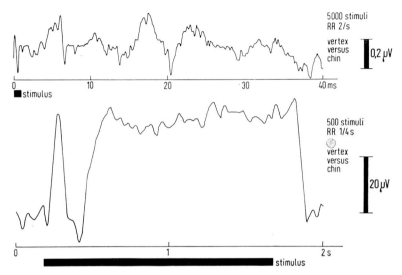

FIG. 5. Simultaneous recording of the response components described above. In place of the 10 millisec scale, a 40 millisec scale was chosen here for the early response; thus, the responses with latencies between 15 and 30 millisec are particularly clear.

comparison with Fig. 4 that Fig. 4 gives better information about N_1 and N_2 and the 6 to 8 millisec response and that Fig. 5, with a 40 milli-sec time scale, gives best insight into the early response with a latency between 15 and 30 millisec.

Up to now we have reported the results obtained by means of the averaging technique. The type of pattern of the responses, especially of the early ones, however, makes it clear that some periodicity of different frequency ranges is embedded in the complex responses. If one skips the time domain and switches to the frequency domain, it is tempting to change the technology from the averaging use of the computer to the correlation function record by means of a fast correlator, as mentioned in the title of the paper.

Since the longest available period in the early responses is clearly in the order of 10 to 30 millisec., and the shortest one, related to the N_1 and N_2 responses as well as to the microphonic potentials, is somewhere around 1 kHz, some careful filtering is necessary to obtain best results with a correlator. As is shown in Fig. 6, by filtering between 60 Hz and

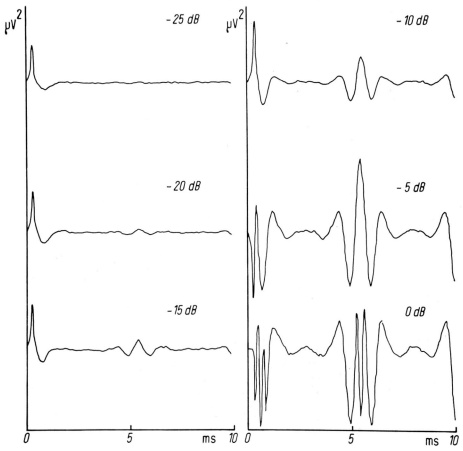

F IG. 6. Autocorrelation function won from the palate recording. (The correlogram should allways start with the highest value at the very beginning but here and also in Figs 7 and 8 this excluded.)

600 Hz both the N_1 and N_2 responses, and the two other early responses around 6 and 10 millisec and around 15 to 30 millisec, can be used for the autocorrelation functions obtainable from the hard palate electrode. In this figure, however, we restricted ourselves to an upper frequency of about 600, although the repetition rate was in the order of 200 stimuli per second down to 100 per second. In the latter case, as is shown in Fig. 6, a time scale of the $\Delta\tau$ of the autocorrelation function of

10 millisec covers the computed time range. Though the frequency of the repetition rate is clearly embedded in the autocorrelation function recorded in Fig. 6 corresponding to 5 millisec. $\Delta\tau$ in this figure, and also, in addition, the quick components embedded in the N_1 and N_2 responses are clearly detectable as fast swings within the autocorrelation function. It should be mentioned that just by the inertia of the xy plotter the very first $\Delta\tau$ is not recorded correctly; it should be the biggest one by far, and it actually is, when looking at the cathode-ray-tube-display of the autocorrelator. In our case we used a Hewlett-Packard correlator type 3721A, which turned out to be very useful for this purpose and if one compares it with the electronic device necessary for a good averaging it is indeed relatively less expensive, maybe by a factor of 10 to 100 as compared with a good averager. So for clinical use it might well be the case that in the future, by omitting the time pattern and by just looking at the detectable records of bioelectrical activities elicited by the sound stimuli described above, the amount of equipment necessary for recording can be drastically reduced. Figure 6 shows clearly that those autocorrelograms related to clicks with increasing intensity increase, too, in a non-linear manner, but begin about 30 dB lower than the threshold for the middle ear muscle reflex activity. It should be mentioned that in Fig. 6 the lower trace, right row, is clipped for the high amplitudes. That the records are not electrical or mechanical artifacts can be proven. Figure 7 shows a comparison between the autocorrelograms obtained at an intensity around 70 dB above threshold before and after adaptation of two

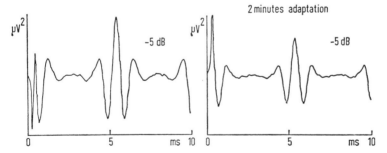

FIG. 7. Comparison between the autocorrelograms obtained at an intensity of about 70 dB above threshold before and after adaptation.

minutes. The figure reveals clearly a decrease in amplitude after adaptation, which could not happen if the records would be artifacts. In addition, if one records the autocorrelation with an open electrical circuit, if there would be any electrical artifact it should be enlarged. As the figure shows, there is no signal on the autocorrelogram at all, with

F

the exception of the effect of the high-pass-ride of the active filter system
at the very beginning, but the correlogram at 5, 10, 15, etc., millisec is
completely gone. To summarize, there can be no doubt that by using
a fast correlator it is possible to record the four early responses simultaneously and with a relatively easily obtainable technological equipment. We therefore believe that this type of record could be of real help
for clinical use in the future, as already stated. On the other hand,
coming back to the topic of the first part of the paper, we would posi-

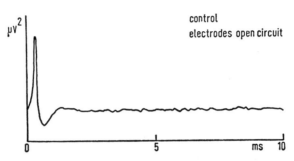

FIG. 8. Control-autocorrelation with an open electrical circuit in order to eliminate artefacts.

tively recommend recording simultaneously from vertex and hard
palate electrode in the future, using the averaging technique in addition
and thus having access to the time domain, too. Recording seven
different events within the entire auditory pathway and thus getting
information from at least five different neuronal levels, the maximum
amount of information available from the different parts of the auditory
channel can be recorded objectively by means of the additional use of a
palate electrode.

REFERENCES

Aran, J. M., Portmann, M., Portmann, Cl. and Pelerin, J. (1970). Electro-
    cochleography in adults and children. Electro-physiological study of the peri-
    pheral receptors. *10th Int. Congr. Audiology, Dallas, Texas* (11–15 Oct., 1970).
David, E., Finkenzellar, P., Kallert, S. and Keidel, W. D. (1969). Interaction
    between visual and auditory evoked de-potentials in man. *In:* Biokybernetik,
    Bd. III; Hnsg. Drischel, H. und N. Tiedt, VEB Gustav Fisher Verlag, Jena,
    1971.
David, E., Finkenzeller, P., Kallert, S. and Keidel, W. D. (1969). Akustischen
    Reizen zugeordnete Gleichspannungsänderungen am intakten Schädel des
    Menschen. *Pflügers Arch.*, **309**, 362–367.
Elberling, C. and Salomon, G. (1970). Ublodig recording af aktionspotentialer fra
    hørenerven. *Nordisk Akustisk Mode, Kopenhagen* (24–26 August, 1970).
Keidel, W. D. (1970a). Some new facts and interpretations in neurophysiology of
    hearing. *Nordisk Akustisk Mode, Kopenhagen* (24–26 August, 1970).

Keidel, W. D. (1970b). Zentrale neurophysiologische Grundmechanismen bei der akustischen Zeichenerkennung des Menschen. IV wissenschaftlichen HNO Tagung der DDR vom 7–10 Okt. 1970 in Halle.

Keidel, W. D. (1971). What do we know about the human cortical evoked potential after all. *Arch. klin. exp. Ohr-Nas. u. Kehl. Heilk.*, **198**, 9–37.

Salomon, G. and Elberling, C. (1970). Elektrisk Response Audiometri på IBM 1800 datamat i klinikken. *Nordisk Akustisk Mode, Kopenhagen* (24–26 August, 1970).

Walter, G. W. (1967). Electrical signs of association expectancy and decision in the human brain. *Electroenceph. clin. Neurophysiol.* Suppl., **25**, 258–263.

Yoshie, N. (1968). Auditory nerve action potential responses to clicks in man. *Laryngoscope*, **78**, 198–215.

Some Aspects of the Audiology of Familial Hearing Loss

I. G. TAYLOR

in collaboration with
V. BRASIER, W. D. HINE, T. MORRIS
AND C. A. POWELL
*Department of Audiology and Education of the Deaf,
The University, Manchester, England*

Fraser (1970) confirms that perhaps a third or more of deaf persons remain without an assigned cause of deafness. He rightly points out that an analysis of this group of unknown causes is a difficult one and presents the main obstacles to establishing even an appropriate aetiological balance sheet. Having pointed out all the difficulties in identifying cause and effect Fraser presents a tentative balance sheet of causation on the 2,355 children of the school study in the British Isles. He estimates that:

Genetically determined deafness accounts for 50·2 per cent of that total—of which 25·4 per cent of that total are cases of clinically un-differentiated autosomal recessive deafness making a total of auto-somal recessive cases 33·2 per cent taking into account the syndromes associated with goitre, retinitis pigmentosia, ECG abnormalities and others.

Fraser's figures for autosomal dominant conditions amount to 15·3 per cent. The figure of 50·2 per cent taken at its face value would indicate the considerable importance played in genetical factors in the causation of familial deafness. It also appears unlikely that the number of children deaf as a result of genetic causes will become less. The immediate hope for a re-education in the number of deaf children appears to lie in the fields of prevention of maternal rubella, kernic-terus, peripnatal disorder and other acquired conditions. Fraser's very interesting approach to the causes of profound deafness in childhood includes a detailed account of the nature of inherited deafness as seen from the point of view of the geneticist.

It would therefore appear from this account by Fraser that the estimate of 25·4 per cent for clinically undifferentiated autosomal recessive deafness and 12·2 per cent for clinically undifferentiated autosomal dominant deafness constitute a considerable portion of the percentage which are usually referred to as "cause unknown".

It appears perfectly reasonable to expect that a considerable proportion of children labelled as "cause unknown" will have a genetic basis as the cause of their deafness. Furthermore, the basis is more likely to be recessive than dominant. In dominant deafness where one parent is deaf or a considerable family history of congenital deafness is known to exist then a dominant genetic basis may be assumed. On the other hand if this condition is recessive then the parents will have normal hearing and if there are other children in the family they also may have normal hearing. In the nature of Mendelian inheritance the chances of each child being deaf is one in four. It may well be that in a recessively inherited deafness in an imaginary family of three children, all three may be deaf or on the other hand two may be deaf and one normal, or one deaf and two normal, or there may be three clinically normal children.

In our present investigation my colleagues and I approached the problem of familial deafness from another angle in order to investigate whether a different but complementary appraisal would help our understanding. Firstly, we looked at one school for deaf children, identifying the causes of deafness in each child from their medical history and examination, and secondly, a study of families when a dominantly inherited deafness was present.

IDENTIFICATION OF GROUPS IN THE SCHOOL

As far as was possible the causes of deafness in the 86 children were assigned as follows:

(i) Familial: 17 children—two or more from the same family, excluding the rh. factor and where examination revealed no other abnormality 17

    4 with one or more deaf parent 4

(ii) Jaundice due to the rh. factor 16

(iii) Anoxia or premature 13

(iv) Rubella (history and also other clinical signs of the disease) 7

(v) Meningitis 5

(vi) Unknown 24

                           TOTAL   86

Audiological measurements made on all these children included:

(i) Pure tones—air and bone threshold measurements.
(ii) Speech audiograms.
(iii) Stapedial reflex thresholds.

The speech audiograms were obtained using the Boothroyd lists.

Stapedial reflex levels were obtained using the Madsen impedance bridge and recording the results using the XY Plotter. Graphic reading of the results is infinitely superior to attempts at readings directly from the dials. Loudness discomfort levels were determined by asking the children to indicate when the sounds became too loud or unpleasant. Little or no difficulty was experienced when the sound became "too loud". Any attempts at finer definition of loudness discomfort seemed pointless. The audiometers used in these experiments have a rise time of 40 millisec.

The reason for determination of the pure tone, stapedial reflex threshold and L.D.L. was to identify in each child whether abnormal loudness function was present or not. In cases of bilateral perceptive deafness where loudness balance tests are not available the determination of the stapedial reflex and the loudness discomfort levels seemed to offer the best method of identification.

For the purpose of this study loudness disorder was judged to be occurring if the span between pure tone and stapedial reflex threshold fell below 65 dB. It was possible to make this measurement when pure tone losses indicated a sensori neural loss and when loudness dysfunction was present. Children were therefore classified as showing loudness dysfunction, *not* showing loudness dysfunction, or indeterminate (because they were too deaf). Loudness discomfort levels have been described by Hood and Poole (1966) in cases of Meniéres disease where loudness dysfunction was known to be present. These workers found that sound pressure levels of 100 dB were unpleasantly loud irrespective of the magnitude of the hearing loss. The reasons for inclusion of the latter test were several, but mainly to give additional evidence of the presence or absence of loudness dysfunction in deaf children when the stapedial reflex was not obtainable and to investigate the value of the test with congenitally deaf children in contrast to the deafened adult with Meniéres disease.

Returning to the group of children in the study the results were as follows for the five groups of so-called "known" causes.

AUDIOGRAMS

The results were subjected to an analysis of variance. The variables of

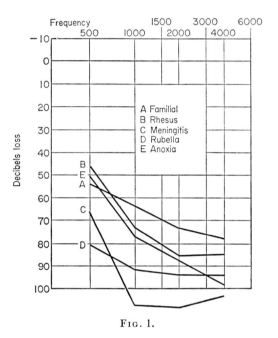

Fig. 1.

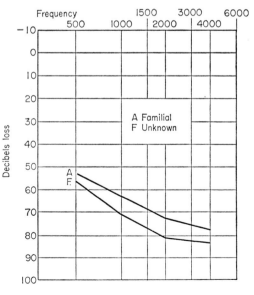

Fig. 2.

interest were the groups and the interaction of groups and frequencies. This latter provided a measure of differences in slope of audiograms among the various groups. The interaction was found to be significant. It was concluded that the audiogram patterns of the five groups differed among themselves. Because of this significant interaction it was not possible to test whether the levels of the mean audiograms differed. It was therefore decided to test the hearing losses of the different groups at 1,000 Hz. These levels were also found to differ among themselves. It seemed reasonable to conclude that there were real differences between both the shapes and the levels of the mean audiograms of the five "known" groups.

The next step was to determine to what extent the mean audiograms for the "unknown" group resembled any of the "known" group. An analysis of variances gives an F value of less than one for the groups—by frequencies interaction. The F value for the hearing loss levels between the familial genetic and the "unknown" group is only just greater than one and this is of course non-significant (Fig. 2).

To summarize, this part, the five aetiological groups differed among themselves both in shape and level. *On the other hand the "unknown" group differs from the familial groups neither in shape nor in level.*

STAPEDIAL REFLEX THRESHOLDS AND ABNORMAL LOUDNESS FUNCTION

A test was made of the distribution of those who did or did not show evidence of loudness disorder or were indeterminate in the familial aetiology group and in the other aetiological groups combined. The numbers were 20 familial cases showing loudness dysfunction and 23 indeterminate among the other aetiologies. χ^2 for this distribution was 17·247 which, with one degree of freedom, is significant at better than 1 per cent level. Finally, the distribution of cases in the familial and the unknown groups were examined. Fisher's exact probability test was used and P was found to be 0·072 indicating that the two groups did not differ significantly in distribution of those showing loudness disorder and those who were indeterminate. The actual figures were 20 familial cases showing evidence of loudness disorder, and one not; 18 unknown showing loudness disorder and 6 indeterminate.

However these findings have to be interpreted with caution. As has already been noted the familial cases had slighter overall hearing losses than the other aetiological groups and were therefore more likely to be testable for loudness disorder while cases from the other aetiological groups had greater losses and were therefore more likely to be classified as indeterminate.

LOUDNESS DISCOMFORT LEVEL

Three groups were compared for loudness discomfort levels. These were the familial cases who showed evidence of loudness disorder (19 out of 21), children from the other aetiological groups who showed evidence of loudness disorder (N = 17) and thirdly children from the other aetiological groups who were too deaf to assess for loudness dysfunction (N = 23). It should be noted that where no discomfort was detected at 130 dB the discomfort level was assumed to be 140 dB, the threshold of pain. An analysis of variance indicated that no difference could be detected in loudness discomfort levels between the three groups, nor was there any detectable difference between the groups in shape across the four frequencies (for both tests F was less than one). However there was strong evidence that for the four groups (the three previously mentioned together with the "unknown" group) as a whole there was a tendency for the loudness discomfort level to fall across the four frequencies measured (F = 10·87 with 3 and 168 degrees of freedom. The probability is considerably less than one in a hundred of such an event occurring by chance). From 500 to 4,000 Hz the loudness discomfort level fell on the average 8 dB. (See accompanying table.)

TABLE I
Pure Tone Means and S.Ds

	N	500	1 k	2 k	4 k
Familial	21	54·3 + 17·8	66·7 + 18·3	73·6 + 17·7	76·7 + 26·5
Rhesus	16	45·6 + 13·0	72·5 + 14·4	85·3 + 21·1	85·3 + 21·7
Mening.	5	68·0 + 24·1	107·0 + 24·9	107·0 + 24·9	105·0 + 25·5
Rubella	7	79·3 + 15·1	90·4 + 14·3	91·4 + 19·5	91·4 + 21·2
Anoxia	12	50·8 + 13·5	67·5 + 9·9	85·4 + 24·0	94·2 + 24·4
Unknown	24	58·3 + 28·4	73·1 + 16·9	80·4 + 21·5	83·1 + 22·6

TABLE II
Loudness Discomfort Levels Means and S.Ds

	N	500	1 k	2 k	4 k
Fam. (abnormal loudness function)	19	122·1 + 13·9	123·2 + 14·7	126·6 + 14·5	126·3 + 16·8
Others „	17	122·1 + 7·7	124·7 + 9·8	131·5 + 9·5	132·4 + 9·4
Others too deaf	23	122·8 + 16·3	127·4 + 12·7	128·5 + 11·9	131·3 + 12·6
Unknown	24	123·5 + 13·9	126·2 + 10·9	130·2 + 10·7	130·6 + 11·1
All groups—excldg. unknown	59	122·3 + 13·3	125·3 + 12·4	128·7 + 12·2	130·0 + 13·4

Unknown: 17 showed evidence of loudness dysfunction out of 24.
Familial: 19 showed evidence of loudness dysfunction out of 21.

It was concluded that loudness discomfort level did not help in determining the presence or otherwise of loudness disorder in this group of children and that the mean loudness discomfort level for this group of children was of the order of 125 dB.

Considerable doubt exists as to the significance of the loudness discomfort determinate as a useful indication of loudness dysfunction particularly in severe congenital deafness. In this series the measure proved to be of little value and certainly not comparable to the stapedial reflex measurements. In our investigation no useful evidence was furnished which would have helped to identify aetiological groups and loudness dysfunction.

The possibilities of combining audiological investigation with genetic studies is indicated by this first study. At this juncture the evidence for the study will need to be deepened and widened to determine whether the evidence of this work can be shown in a larger study. The methodology used in this study indicates that further work is feasible.

FAMILY STUDIES WHERE THE NATURE OF THE GENETIC INHERITANCE APPEARS TO BE DOMINANT

Three families were studied to investigate the variation which may exist amongst the various members of the same family.

Family No. 1

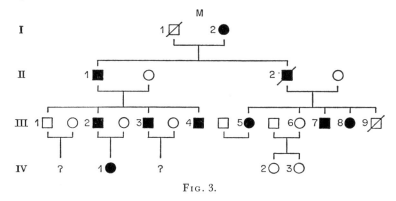

FIG. 3.

It will be seen that there are two main branches to this family. An analysis of variance was undertaken of the audiograms of the deaf members of the two branches of the family. Losses at three frequencies in the better ear were considered. The interaction between the groups and frequencies was found to be insignificant. The F value for the group was

16·39 which, with 1 and 5 degrees of freedom, was significant at beyond the 1 per cent level. It was concluded that the two branches of the family differ in degree of hearing loss in the better ear.

	k/Hz			
	250	1 k	4 k	N
Branch A	26·7	45·0	43·3	3
Branch B	51·2	67·5	80·0	4

An analysis of variance was undertaken of the stapedial reflexes of the deaf and normally hearing members of this family. Two groups (deaf and normally hearing) and two frequencies (better ear 1 kHz and 2 kHz) were considered. The interaction between groups and frequencies was not significant $(F < 1)$. The F value for groups was 8·99 which is significant at better than the 5 per cent level. It was concluded that the mean stapedial reflex level for the deaf group was greater than that for the hearing group at the 1 kHz and 2 kHz.

	1 k	2 k	N
Deaf	97·9	100·7	7
Normal	88·3	90·0	6

The study of this family showed that there can be considerable differences in hearing loss (Fig. 4 and Fig. 5) in different branches of

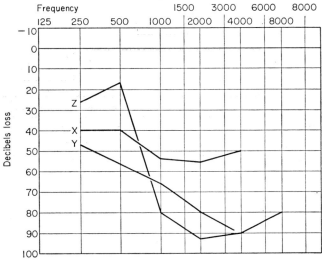

FIG. 4. Pure tone audiograms.

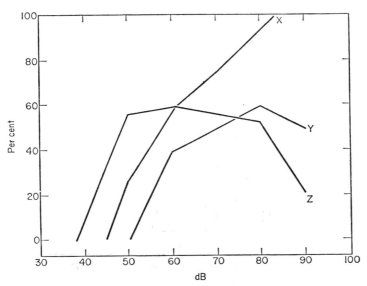

FIG. 5. Speech audiograms.

the same family and that those differences, as in this family, may result in different educational management. The deafer branch of the family attended a school for the deaf whilst the other group attended ordinary school.

Family No. 2

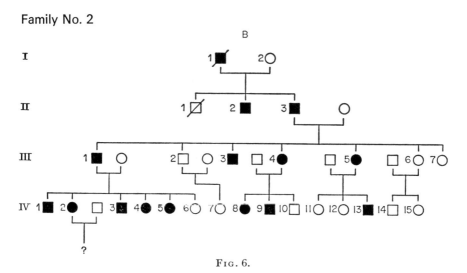

FIG. 6.

Three branches formed this family. The means and standard deviations of audiograms of Ba, Be and A are given below:

	N	·5	1 k	2 k	4 k
Ba	6	29·2 ± 15·9	50·0 ± 24·1	80·0 ± 21·2	80·0 ± 16·6
Be	2	45·0 ± 7·1	57·5 ± 10·6	67·5 ± 17·7	67·5 ± 31·8
A	3	53·3 ± 7·6	60·0 ± 8·7	83·3 ± 5·8	95·0 ± 5·0

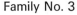

Family No. 3

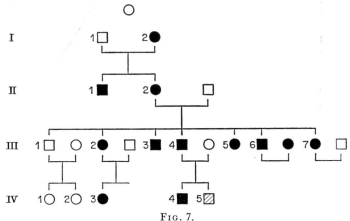

FIG. 7.

This family is listed as "O" under the means and standard deviations of all audiograms:

O	6	56·7 ± 15·7	64·2 ± 19·9	70·0 ± 22·4	65·8 ± 24·8

An analysis of variance showed that the three branches of Family No. 2 do not differ in shape or level of audiogram. There is as much difference within the branches as between them ($F = 1·08$ for shape, $F = 1·06$ for level), but it will be understood that the individual variations are of considerable significance in educational placement and management.

RECESSIVE AND DOMINANT FAMILIES

Comparisons were made between the mean audiograms of deaf members of dominant and recessive families. As the numbers in the recessive families were small it was decided to combine these cases. There were thus four groups, including deaf subjects from three recessive families and the other three consisting of deaf members of three dominant families.

A significant F value was found for slope of audiogram ($F = 5·24$ with 9 and 81 degrees of freedom, the probability of such a high value of F occurring by chance being less than one in a hundred). Inspection seemed to indicate that this was due to Family A, whose mean audiogram showed a steep slope falling 45 dB from 500 to 4,000 Hz. Although the mean audiograms of the other families also fell across these frequencies they did so at a much smaller rate (e.g. recessives fell 7 dB; M family 20 dB; O family 9 dB). It was concluded that recessive and dominant families cannot be distinguished from one another by means of their mean audiogram slope and that indeed the dominant families differ among themselves in mean audiogram slope. Numbers of members of recessive families were too small to make a test of differences between recessive families possible.

TABLE III
Dominant Families (Deaf)

	Loudness Dysfunction (<65)	Unknown
Bar.	7	2
M	7	–
O	5	–

Recessive

	Loudness Dysfunction	Unknown
T.	3	–
H.	1	1
S.	–	2

The subjects were classified as showing loudness dysfunction if the span between the pure tone and stapedial reflex threshold at any frequency was less than 65 dB. The presence or absence of loudness dysfunction is unknown for all others. The question of dividing this group into those definitely not showing loudness dysfunction was considered, the proposed method being to classify those with a loss greater than 35 dB but less than 55 dB at any frequency as no loudness dysfunction if the stapedial reflex were absent. However this method was considered invalid as on this basis five subjects known to be recruiting would have been classified as non-recruiting.

STAPEDIAL

All the families showed evidence of recruitment in one or other member except in one instance. However their hearing levels are too severe to necessarily expect a reflex.

Levels of Stapedial Reflex in Normals (Spans)

In the dominant group, of the ten subjects tested, all showed reflexes at a pathological level as defined in the paper, on either ear at any frequency. Only four subjects gave no sign of an abnormal reflex on either ear, two were borderline pathological on the low side, and four were borderline high (2) or absent (2). The mean span at each frequency was as follows for the better ear:

500 Hz	1,000 Hz	2,000 Hz	4,000 Hz
84	85	87	84 dB

For the recessive group, of the six subjects tested, five subjects showed a reflex span within the normal range, but for one subject no reflex could be obtained. The number that showed no evidence of a pathological span on either ear was two, for the other four the span was on the high side. The mean spans of the reflexes that could be obtained is as follows for the better ear:

500 Hz	1,000 Hz	2,000 Hz	4,000 Hz
92	88	94	92dB

Levels of Stapedial Reflex in Normals

In the dominant group all the subjects showed stapedial reflexes within the normal range at some frequencies. If 70–95 dB is taken as normal then four subjects had all reflexes within this range and five subjects showed reflexes that were higher than this.

The mean levels were:

500 Hz	1,000 Hz	2,000 Hz	4,000 Hz
93·5	89	91	90·5dB

In the recessive group, three of the six subjects tested showed reflexes within the normal range at some frequencies; for the other three the level was high. Four of the subjects had high reflexes for some frequencies only two being within the normal range for them all.

The mean levels were:

500 Hz	1,000 Hz	2,000 Hz	4,000 Hz
95	91	102	87dB

CONCLUSIONS

This investigation is concerned with the detailed study of 86 hearing impaired children. Comparisons are made between the different audiological findings in the different aetiological groups. Significant differences were found in the mean pure tone audiogram shape amongst the five groups where causation of deafness was identifiable. There were no significant differences found between the familial genetic and the unknown group.

Stapedial reflex thresholds and loudness discomfort thresholds indicated in this study that stapedial reflex measurements did give evidence of the presence of loudness disorder in certain groups of children. The use of loudness discomfort measurement proved to be disappointingly negative in all cases. Care has been taken at this stage not to equate abnormal loudness function as defined in the study with the classical loudness recruitment.

This investigation of children does highlight the limitation of classical tests of loudness recruitment in paediatric audiology and emphasizes the need to continue to study the effects of cochlea pathology in congenital and acquired lesions.

The most significant finding is the almost complete identification of the pure tone audiogram of the genetic familial group with the "unknown" group. It is too early to make any final conclusion on the significance of this finding until further studies have been made. It is to be noted that this report would give some further support to the view that many of the children whose causes of deafness are recorded as "unknown" are, in fact, deafened as a result of a genetically inherited factor.

The family studies of the dominant inherited type indicates the individual variations in different branches of the same family and the educational consequences which may result.

Comparisons of audiological findings of the "dominant" and "recessive" families did not indicate any way of recognizing differences by any known audiological technique.

ACKNOWLEDGEMENTS

Special thanks must be given to Mr Furness and his staff, at the School for the Partially Hearing, Southport, who supplied a great deal of important information on all the children and who made special provision for our testing procedures.

Mr Hine undertook the statistical analysis of the material.

REFERENCES

Fraser, G. R. (1970). "The Causes of Profound Deafness in Childhood." 5–40. Ciba Foundation Symposia, 1970. J. & A. Churchill, London.

Hood, J. D. and Poole, J. P. (1966). Tolerable limit of loudness: its clinical and physiological significance. *J. acoust. Soc. Am.*, **40**, 47–53.

G

The Role of the Auditory Cortex in Sound Localization

I. C. WHITFIELD

Neurocommunications Research Unit,
University of Birmingham, Birmingham, England

The ability to localize sound depends to a substantial extent upon the possession of two ears. Because sound travels at a finite speed, a sound on the left will reach the left ear before it reaches the right ear, and because of the shadowing effect of the head it will, in general, be louder in the left ear than the right. However, this cannot be the whole answer, because we can locate sounds in elevation as well as in azimuth, and even do so with one ear, although the results are not so accurate. Indeed, when we look more closely we find that differential time of arrival is a rather ambiguous clue, as there are many possible positions of the source that give the same time differential.

The difference in time of arrival between the two ears is something like 500 μsec in man when the sound is right over on one side of the head. Suppose we try to imitate this by putting on a pair of ear-phones and presenting a pair of clicks, one to each ear. As we alter the time interval between them from $+ 500$ μsec through zero to $- 500$ μsec the sound image certainly moves, but it seems to move inside our heads rather than out in space. This again suggests there may be more to sound localization than just time difference. One such element is the frequency spectrum. Different frequency components in a signal undergo different degrees of attenuation at the two ears as a result of the influence of the head and the pinnae, and it seems that the resulting information can be utilized, much as in vision we use such things as parallax, and the change of colour produced by atmospheric absorption, to assess distance.

Clearly, if time disparity $(\varDelta t)$ is important, the time difference must be assessed at some point, and we can study the physiology of this process by the paired-click method. The first level at which inputs from the two ears can interact is at the superior olive and we find indeed that some cells at this level are sensitive to $\varDelta t$. The probability of response of cells in the medial superior olive is a function of Δt, and of the differential intensity ΔI at the two ears (Hall, 1965). It is also of course a function of the overall intensity but whereas changes in Δt or ΔI change the probability of firing in opposite directions in the two nuclei (left and right), change in the mean intensity changes the probabilities in the *same* direction. Thus the important clue is the difference between the activities on the two sides. This differential activity passes upwards in the lateral lemnisci and is processed at a higher level which appears to involve the cortex.

Neff *et al.* (1956) showed that bilateral ablation of the whole auditory cortex resulted in almost total loss of the ability of a cat to localize sound in space, but since then the relationship between the roles of the brain-stem and higher centres has been examined in more detail.

I have already indicated that a click presented to the left ear followed 500 μsec later by a click presented to the right ear sounds to us like a single click in the left ear (and, of course, vice versa for a right-left pair). The same appears to be true for the cat. If we train a cat to make one response to a click in the left ear and a different response to a click in the right ear, it will subsequently treat the LR pair as a click on the left and the RL pair as a click on the right. (Masterton *et al.*, 1967.) It does this immediately without any further training. It "transfers" as we say.

However, the cat without auditory cortex does not do this. Although it too can be trained to give one response to a click in the left ear and another to a click in the right ear (hence it is not deaf) it no longer treats the LR and RL pairs as equivalent to single sounds on the left or right. This suggests that the cortex is necessary in order to mediate the spatial quality of such sounds.

Just as the medial superior olivary nucleus appears to mediate position judgements based on Δt, so the pathway through the lateral nucleus of the superior olive appears to mediate, amongst other things, position judgements based on differences in frequency spectrum, and it is possible, by differential brain stem lesions, to dissociate these two mechanisms to some extent. However, again they come together at the cortex and cortical destruction abolishes both.

It is to be noted that to achieve these results we have to remove both left and right auditory cortices. If we remove only one cortex then the transfer is not impaired. Indeed not only can this somewhat artificial problem be solved, but the animal can localize single sounds in real space, for all practical purposes as well as a normal cat (Neff *et al.*, 1956), The two cortices seem equivalent in this respect—it doesn't matter which one we remove. However, before concluding that the second cortex is redundant for localization let us look at another aspect of the real localization situation.

We have been saying, so far, that a sound source in space produces a signal at one ear, followed some microseconds later by a signal in the other ear. However, this is really only true in the open air, or in an anechoic chamber. In an ordinary room a great deal of sound is reflected from the walls, and reaches the listener several *milliseconds* after the original sound. These reflections are not suppressed, they add to the loudness (which is why a voice is less clearly heard in the open air than in a room); yet all the sound *appears* to come from the speaker's mouth. Why is it that these reflections do not upset the localization?

We can imitate the situation artificially, by setting up two loud-speakers one on the right and one on the left in an anechoic chamber. If now we have a tone pulse on the left speaker followed say 5 millisec later by a similar tone pulse on the right speaker, the combination sounds like a single pulse on the left (and vice versa for the RL case). Note that this is different from the previous case where one sound reached one ear and the other sound the other ear. Here *both* sounds reach *both* ears. Suppose now we teach a cat to go down the left arm of a Y-maze when the left speaker alone is on and down the right arm when the right speaker alone is on (Cranford *et al.*, 1971). If when it has learned this we present "left-before-right" with a 5 millisec interval, this will immediately be treated as if it were a single left, and similarly "right-before-left' will be treated as if it were a single right. This is also, of course, how they appear to humans (Wallach *et al.*, 1949). Suppose now we remove the auditory cortex on only one side (right or left). The cats will still, as we noted earlier, be able to localize the single left or single right speaker, but how about the pairs?

A difficulty in testing animals behaviourally is that if they fail, they run to either side at random and it is difficult to determine whether they have failed as a result of the lesion, or just "given up". We therefore trained the animals before surgery to go left to L-before-R and right to R-before-L as already noted, but we also trained them to go right if presented with an R and L stimulus in which neither was first (they were variable). After surgery we found that the cats with left lesions did LR correctly and the cats with right lesions did RL correctly. However the right lesion cats went to the *right* on LR, showing that this signal had apparently now no sidedness. The left lesion cats also went to the right on RL, but this of course throws no light on the matter, since this is both the correct response to RL and also the correct response if this stimulus had no sidedness. We therefore now reversed the training of these animals to go *left* when the stimulus had no sidedness. The result was that the left lesion animals now tended to go left to RL (which is the "wrong" side), and the right lesion cats stopped going right to LR and were now about neutral. The response of the left lesion cats to LR and of the right lesion cats to RL was substantially unaffected. We conclude therefore that the contralateral cortex is essential for the proper localization of a source under echoic, but not under anechoic conditions. These results may explain the conflicting statements in the literature about the effect of temporal lobe damage on the ability of patients to localize sounds on the side contralateral to the lesion.

REFERENCES

Cranford, J., Ravizza, R., Diamond, I. T. and Whitfield, I. C. (1971). Unilateral ablation of the auditory cortex in the cat impairs complex sound localization. *Science*, **172**, 286–288.

Hall, J. L. (1965). Binaural interaction in the accessory superior-olivary nucleus of the cat. *J. acoust. Soc. Am.*, **37**, 814–823.

Masterton, B., Jane, J. A. and Diamond, I. T. (1967). Role of brainstem auditory structures in sound localization. I. Trapezoid body, superior olive and lateral lemniscus. *J. Neurophysiol.*, **30**, 341–359.

Neff, W. D., Fisher, J. F., Diamond, I. T. and Yela, M. (1956). Role of auditory cortex in discrimination requiring localization of sound in space. *J. Neurophysiol.*, **19**, 500–512.

Wallach, H., Newman, E. B. and Rosenzweig, M. R. (1949). The precedence effect in sound localization. *Am. J. Psychol.*, **62**, 315–336.

The Destructive Effect of Intense Pure Tones on the Cochleae of Mammals

A. PYE

*The Institute of Laryngology and Otology,
London, England*

INTRODUCTION

High intensity sound is known to produce either temporary or permanent damage to the cochlea, both in man and in animals. Since experimental studies in man are restricted to the production of temporary threshold shifts, animals have to be used to demonstrate permanent damage to the cochlea.

Low frequency sounds are analysed towards the apex of the cochlea and high frequencies at the base, although the latter are much more compressed at the basal end. The pattern of this frequency analysis along the basilar membrane also varies in different species of animals. Two preliminary studies, one using the guinea-pig *Procavia* and the other a fruit-bat *Rousettus*, have already been carried out and the work was reported last year Pye (1971).

MATERIAL AND METHODS

The guinea-pig is the most frequently used laboratory animal for experimentally produced acoustic trauma and has been used, among other workers by Davis *et al.* (1953), Eldredge and Covell (1958), Stockwell *et al.* (1969) and Poche *et al.* (1969). In the present study high intensity pure tones were used on the guinea-pig, so as to obtain a narrow spectrum of damage. Frequencies from 4 kHz to 25 kHz were used, as earlier workers had concentrated on lower frequencies and my own previous results indicated that hardly any damage could be obtained above 25 kHz. These pure tones were produced by a sonic-ultrasonic generator (built at the Institute) and an Ionophane 601 loudspeaker. A short flared horn with a 2·5 cm square aperture was used instead of the

89

large exponential horn normally fitted, as the main interest was for the production of intense high frequencies. The maximum intensities, limited by the apparatus, were measured by a Bruel and Kjoer 6·4 mm microphone at 1 cm from the sound source in dB SPL, i.e. dB re 0·00002 N.m^{-2} as follows:

4 kHz	120 dB
8, 10 and 12 kHz	126 dB
15 kHz	125 dB
20 kHz	124 dB
25 kHz	122 dB

These intensities correspond to those used in the earlier experiments (Pye, 1971). The guinea-pigs were restricted in a crush-cage, so that little movement of the head was allowed and only the left ear was exposed (1 cm from the horn), the right ear being used as a control.

For frequencies other than 25 kHz, a 30-min exposure was found to be the optimum time to produce damage, while exposures of at least seven hours were needed to produce damage to the cochlea at 25 kHz. The number of animals used at each frequency was six, except for 10 kHz, where the data for one animal are missing, as the last animal had to be discarded owing to otitis media.

Method of Assessing Damage

High intensity sound causes destruction of the sensory (hair) cells of the cochlea and the best method of assessing damage was developed by Engström *et al.* (1966). This is a quick and reliable method and can be accomplished in a day for each cochlea. The animals are sacrificed three to four weeks after the end of the experiment, so that destruction to the sensory cells has had time to develop. The cochlea is fixed in a buffered solution of osmic acid (1·3 per cent) for two to four hours immediately after killing the animal. The cochlea is then washed in water and dehydrated up to 70 per cent alcohol, where it may be stored for a while. However, it was found best to continue with the dissection on the following day. The cochlea is then micro-dissected, the spiral organ is mounted on slides in glycerine and observed in surface view under phase contrast. The sensory cells are usually arranged in a regular reticular pattern (Fig. 1) and if a cell has been destroyed, it is possible to identify it as a "phalangeal" scar (Fig. 2).

Results

The extent of the damaged area of sensory cells is governed by the duration of the exposure and the location of the damage depends

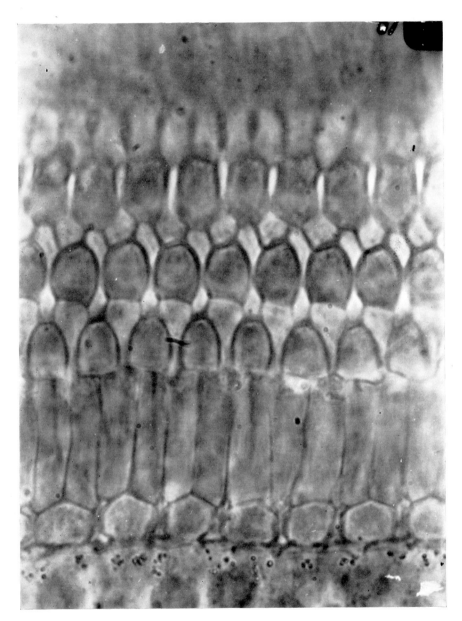

FIG. 1. Surface view of the spiral organ in the guinea-pig viewed under phase contrast. One row of inner sensory cells and the reticular pattern formed by the three rows of outer sensory cells in seen, separated by the pillar cells ($\times$ 1460).

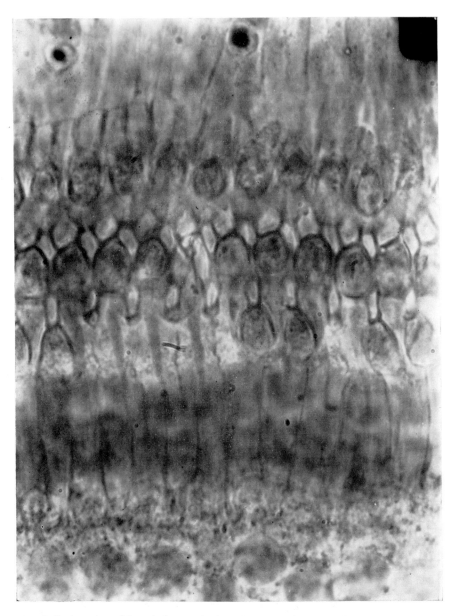

FIG. 2. Surface view of the spiral organ in the guinea-pig, which has been exposed to intense pure tones (end of second turn). The inner row of sensory cells can just be seen. In the outer sensory cells, the innermost row has five cells missing, the middle row shows a "phalangeal" scar and the outermost row is complete. The damage shown here is small and at an edge of a more damaged area ($\times$ 1460).

on the frequencies used. There appears, however, to be a complex relationship between the intensity of the sound and the duration of the exposure.

The guinea-pig has four and a quarter turns to the cochlea and the damage obtained for frequencies used has been mapped out in Table I. Since in no case was the damage less than one-eighth of *any* turn, it was

TABLE I

Damaged Areas in the Cochleae of Guinea-pigs After Exposure to Intense Pure Tones

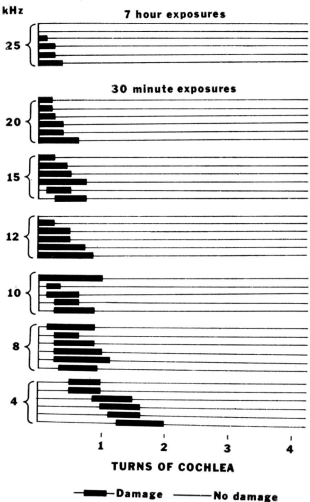

Two different time exposures are given. The damage becomes less widespread and is nearer to the base for higher frequencies.

thought sufficient to observe the extent of the damage by the divisions of the various turns, rather than by counting all the damaged sensory cells, as done by Stockwell *et al.* (1969) and others.

The location of the damage was most variable at 4 kHz; the six animals showed damage which ranged from a point centred at three-quarters of a turn from the base to beyond one and a half turns, although for a single animal the extent of the damage did not exceed three-quarters of a turn. This is comparable with the results of Stockwell *et al.* (1969) whose major area of damage for 4 kHz was from a half turn from the base to the second turn, although minor damage extended throughout the cochlea. These workers used 130 dB SPL intensity at 4 kHz and one hour as their exposure time. By halving the exposure time and using less intense sounds it was hoped to obtain a more restricted area of damage, which, in fact, proved to be the case.

The general trend was that towards the basal (high frequency) part of the cochlea, the extent of the damage becomes less and is least at 25 kHz. No damage could be detected in two animals exposed to that frequency for seven hours or in one animal exposed for 30 min at 12 kHz. Generally, except for one animal at 10 kHz, the damage does not reach the base of the cochlea for frequencies below 12 kHz, but even this is not consistent (see two animals exposed to 15 kHz).

The pattern of damage is as follows: no damage was found to the inner row of sensory cells, but probably higher frequencies are needed to produce that (see Stockwell *et al.*, 1969) at 130 dB. In the partially damaged areas of the outer sensory cells, the middle row was usually damaged most, followed by the outermost and then the innermost rows. In severely damaged areas all the outer sensory cells were destroyed and replaced by "phalangeal" scars. On either side of a completely damaged area there was a region where only slight damage occurred (Fig. 2).

In no case was any damage found in the control ears, except for the irregularities which occur during development at the apex of the cochlea in most animals and which are not attributable to sound exposure.

DISCUSSION

In agreement with other workers there is variability in the damage produced to the spiral organ, both in the extent and severity of it at different frequencies. This suggests that, apart from experimental error and although all the parameters are kept the same, some individuals are more sensitive to sound than others.

CONCLUSIONS

These results indicate that permanent damage to the cochlea generally occurred in the guinea-pig after only 30 min exposure to intense pure tones, although some frequencies (e.g. 25 Hz) required exposure time as long as seven hours. The damaged area can be restricted to give a more precise result by choosing the shortest time of exposure to produce damage at a given frequency. The next phase of this work will concern itself with the finding of the optimum intensity.

These results also agree with the physiological findings by cochlear microphonics of many workers (the latest Dallos et al., 1970), who mapped out the frequency analysis pattern of the cochlea in the guinea-pig. They found that local responses up to 10 kHz can be measured from the basal turn, up to 3 kHz in the second turn and up to 500 Hz in the third turn.

The implications of the present study on the hearing of human beings could be manyfold: permanent damage to the cochlea might be induced within short periods of exposure to any form of industrial noise, if the sound intensities are high enough.

It is hoped to continue this study by monitoring cochlear microphonic responses from externally placed electrodes with the use of a lock-in amplifier following Brown et al. (1970). After sound exposure experiments the electrodes could be placed in position and cochlear microphonics recorded at various frequencies and time intervals for comparison with normal responses. It is also hoped to extend this study on experimental acoustic trauma to other animals, whose frequency ranges are different from that of the guinea-pig, so that more knowledge may be gained into the physiology of hearing.

ACKNOWLEDGEMENTS

Thanks are due to: Mr W. A. Gray of the Institute of Laryngology and Otology, who built the sonic-ultrasonic generator, Mr D. J. Connolly of the Department of Clinical Photography of the Institute of Laryngology and Otology, for the reproduction of the illustrations. This research was sponsored by the Wellcome Trust.

REFERENCES

Brown, K. S., Gordon, B. and Cavonius, C. R. (1970). Microphonic potentials from the skin predict inner ear defects in cats. Nature, Lond., **228**, 1212.

Dallos, P., Schveny, Z. G. and Cheatham, M. A. (1970). On the limitations of cochlear-microphonic measurements. J. acoust Soc. Am., **49**, 1144.

Davis, H., Benson, R. W., Covell, W. P., Fernandez, C., Goldstein, R., Katsuki, Y., Legouix, J. P., McAulisse, D. R. and Tasaki, I. (1953). Acoustic trauma in the guinea-pig. J. acoust Soc. Am., **25**, 1180.

Eldredge, D. H. and Covell, W. P. (1958). A laboratory method for the study of acoustic trauma in the guinea-pig. Laryngol., **68**, 465.

Engström, H., Ades, H. W. and Andersson, A. (1966). "The Structural Pattern of the Organ of Corti". Almqvist and Wiksell, Stockholm.

Poche, L. B., Stockwell, C. W. and Ades, H. W. (1969). Cochlear hair cells damage in guinea-pigs after exposure to impulse noise. *J. acoust Soc. Am.*, **46**, 947.

Pye, A. (1971). Effect of exposure to intense pure tones on the hearing organ of animals. *Rev. Acustica*, **II**, 199–203.

Stockwell, C. W., Ades, H. W. and Engström, E. (1969). Patterns of hair cell damage after intense auditory stimulation. *Ann. Otol. Rhinol. Laryngol.*, **78**, 1144.

Electrical Traveling Waves in the Chinchilla Cochlea

D. H. ELDREDGE, L. D. BENITEZ*
and J. W. TEMPLER**

Central Institute for the Deaf, St Louis, Missouri, U.S.A.

INTRODUCTION

In 1952 Tasaki *et al.* described a method for recording cochlear microphonic voltages (CM) with differential electrodes in the cochlea of the guinea-pig. The voltage difference between one electrode in scala vestibuli and a second electrode in scala tympani showed a graded potential that was a low-pass filtered version of the acoustic signal measured as a function of time. This CM was free of whole-nerve action potential and appeared to reflect the voltage arising from a length of the basilar membrane one millimeter either side of the electrodes. When the CM responses from each of the four turns of the guinea-pig cochlea were compared two important differences were observed. First, the responses showed successive delays from base to apex. Secondly, the upper-frequency limit of the low-pass filtering was high near the base and became successively lower toward the apex. Both of these features were consistent with the Békésy traveling wave.

Later Teas *et al.* (1962), showed that it was possible to reconstruct spatial voltage gradients at successive temporal intervals from CM recorded at each of the four turns of the cochlea of guinea-pig. To the extent that CM does reflect displacement of the basilar membrane as demonstrated by von Békésy (1951), this also seemed a good way to demonstrate the Békésy traveling wave. Teas *et al.*, prepared a short film of the electrical traveling waves in response to two low-frequency clicks or thumps that had relatively simple acoustic and CM waveforms. The results were satisfactory but led to more speculation. What happens when this method is applied to other signals? Does the result lead to some better insight concerning the peripheral processes involved in

* Now at Department of Physiology, Ciudad University, Mexico City.
** Now at Denver, Colorado.

frequency discrimination or the tuning of individual primary auditory neurons to narrow ranges of frequencies? For these reasons we decided to extend the observations of Teas *et al.*

Many people have noted the discrepancies between the broad maximum in the envelope of the Békésy traveling wave and the high degree of tuning to a narrow band of frequencies shown by single fibers in the auditory nerve. Others have noted the discrepancy between the Békésy envelope and the very small auditory difference limen for tonal frequency. For example, Huggins and Licklider (1951) discussed this problem and suggested several schemes for mechanical sharpening. These included derivatives of amplitude in both space and time. Some of our unpublished observations suggest that nerve action potentials relate better to rate of change in CM than to amplitude of CM. For this reason we chose to emphasize the derivative with respect to time. Once we had completed our new observations on the amplitudes of the electrical traveling wave, we found it relatively easy to construct additional gradients that approximate the first derivatives of the CM voltage with respect to time as functions of space and at successive times. Animations of the spatial gradients of these derivatives were examined for spatial or temporal sharpening that might correspond to the sharpening implied by the neural response areas. Also many studies of the responses of single auditory neurons indicate enhancement of the probability of neural responses during one half of the period of a tone and suppression of the probability of responses during the other half. Some unpublished studies done at Central Institute for the Deaf suggest, for CM recorded as described above, that the half-cycle for enhancement begins at the time scala vestibuli begins to go negative with respect to scala tympani. For the film enhancement also began when scala vestibuli started negative and the magnitude of the enhancement was proportional to the rate of change of CM voltage.

METHODS

The basic methods were essentially identical to those reported much earlier by Tasaki *et al.* (1952) and by Teas *et al.* (1962). However, we chose the chinchilla as an experimental animal because it was being used in other behavioral and physiological studies of hearing in our laboratories. Differential electrodes were placed across each of the three cochlear turns to record three spatially independent samples of CM. Twenty responses to each signal were averaged on a LINC computer in order to achieve better signal-to-noise ratios in the responses at low sound pressures. The acoustic signals were: (1) a filtered click with major energy at frequencies below 650 Hz and quite similar to those used earlier by Teas *et al.*; (2) a wide-band click generated by leading a 0·1 msec electrical square wave to a dynamic ear-phone (PDR-10) sealed to the external auditory meatus through a tight-fitting speculum, and with significant acoustic energy out nearly to 10 kHz; and (3) short tone pulses at 150 Hz, 500 Hz, and 2,000 Hz. Each onset and decay was three cycles and these bounded plateaus of two, three and four cycles from lowest to highest frequency, respectively.

The locations of the pairs of differential electrodes along the cochlear partition were 3·2, 9·3, and 13·4 mm from the round window end of the basilar membrane as measured on cochlear reconstructions from sections of celloidin-embedded temporal bones. The voltages for each positive and negative peak in the CM waveforms at each place were measured and plotted as functions of distance from the round window. Then a spatial envelope for each peak was made by extrapolating smoothly from zero at the round window end through each measured point to another zero at the apparent apical end. Similar spatial envelopes for the guinea-pig were shown in Fig. 5 of Teas *et al.* (1962).

After the voltage at each place for a peak was established by the envelope it was also necessary to find when the peak reached each place. A peak was identified on each of the three CM functions and the time that the peak arrived at each recording site was measured. These data were plotted on space-time coordinates similar to Fig. 6 of Teas *et al.*, and, from the slopes established by the measurements, smoothed functions were interpolated and extrapolated to describe the times at which the peak reached all places. Similar functions were drawn for the onset of CM and for each zero-crossing as well as for each peak.

Final reconstruction of the spatial voltage gradients at successive temporal intervals was accomplished in the following way. At any given time there were three measured voltages at three corresponding places that could be plotted as a function of distance along the basilar membrane. The locations of the onset and each peak and zero-crossing were then read from the space-time plots of distinctive features and onset and the zero-crossings were plotted as zeros at the appropriate places. The value for each peak at its appropriate place was read from the voltage envelope as a function of distance and plotted accordingly. This procedure yielded an array of up to 11 measured and inferred voltages as a function of distance, through which a continuous spatial voltage gradient could be interpolated. The procedure was repeated at successive temporal intervals to obtain a series of these gradients similar to those shown in Fig. 7 of Teas *et al.* This series of gradients was then photographed one at a time and projected as a motion picture to show the electrical traveling waves. To approximate the first derivative of CM

H

with respect to time as a function of space we measured the negative-going voltage differences between successive pairs of voltage gradients in space. These values were plotted for each interval between successive traces, photographed, and then projected to show the postulated wave of stimulation.

RESULTS AND CONCLUSIONS

In a written report it is not possible to demonstrate the dynamic properties of the electrical traveling waves and of the progression of the postulated neural-enhancing phases as they appeared on the film. However, it is possible to list some of the characteristics that were observed and to note that the electrical traveling waves were quite consistent with the mechanical traveling waves that Békésy had observed.

For the low-frequency click the major period of the transient response was long compared to the traveling wave delay between the first and second turns. This led to a relatively long in-phase portion of the wave and to an enhancing phase that extended for as much as 60 per cent of the length of the basilar membrane. A similarly long suppressing phase and then a second enhancing phase followed. Even though there was little acoustic energy present in this signal at frequencies above 650 Hz, the CM wave was very broadly distributed from the base to a point apical to the electrodes in the third cochlear turn.

For the wide-band click the waveforms at each recording site were very different. The gross or principal periods for the transient responses in the first, second and third turns were about 0·3 msec, 1·0 msec and 2·5 msec respectively. These reflect a spatial gradient in which the responses to the acoustic energy for a wide band of frequencies are "sorted" and continuously distributed along the basilar membrane with those for higher frequencies towards the base and those for the lower frequencies towards the apex. The period of the enhancing phase as it moves along is comparable to the travelling wave delays. This leads to a short length of enhancing phase which rapidly sweeps along about two-thirds of the length of the basilar membrane. This is closely followed by a suppressing phase, then a second enhancing phase. On the film one can easily see the two enhancing phases "chasing" along the length of the basilar membrane. Both the spatial envelope of CM voltage and the magnitude of the postulated enhancing phase grew as the wave progressed from the base out to about two-thirds of the length of the basilar membrane and then decayed abruptly.

For the tone pip at 150 Hz the CM voltages increased from the first to the second to the third turns. During the two-cycle plateau the waveform in the second turn barely lags that at the base and the phase lag grows to only about 30° at the third turn. In the film the "in-phase" spatial pattern tends to dominate but the "out-of-phase" traveling pattern is also clearly present.

For the tone pip at 500 Hz the CM in the second turn was the largest and the phase lags were about 180° and 360° in the second and third turns respectively. At this frequency the film shows the expected pattern for the traveling waves very clearly. At 2,000 Hz the responses in the first turn are clearly larger than in the second, and no component at 2,000 Hz is recognizable in the third turn. However, the CM in the third turn does show a slow wave that is consistent with a delayed envelope of the tone pip. The phase lag for the response in the second turn was more than 360° and the animation showed very pronounced traveling waves.

Even though the spatial patterns described above were distinctively different, each was broad and each was represented by significant voltages in the first turn. If neural responses were somehow proportional to CM voltages or to displacement of the basilar membrane, then a neuron attached to the place of maximum response to tones at 2,000 Hz also ought to be only slightly less sensitive to tones at 500 Hz and 150 Hz. This does not appear to be true for such units when their tuning curves are measured in terms of an increase in rate of responses to tones. For the tone pip at 500 Hz the animation of the spatial distribution and progression of the rate of change of negative-going CM voltage was also a broad pattern and did not present any clue to the mechanism for neural sharpening.

These electrical traveling waves were observed for tones at 40–55 dB SPL. The one really firm conclusion supported by an exercise of the kind necessary to make the film is that the Békésy traveling wave is clearly present at physiological sound pressures and is not an artifact associated with the very high sound pressures used for the original visual observations. It is easier to comprehend the complexities of the space-time patterns of these traveling waves on the film than on any set of static representations. But viewing the film still leaves some major questions. It seems logically necessary that some aspect of the motion of the traveling wave on the membrane plays a causal role in the process of neural excitation. If these CM voltages accurately reflect the displacements along the basilar membrane, then the nature of the links or steps from basilar membrane motion to excitation of the primary neurons remains obscure. CM can either be one of these links or a physiological epiphenomenon. So far the evidence is not decisive.

ACKNOWLEDGEMENTS

Supported by Research Grant NS 03856 from the National Institute of Neurological Diseases and Stroke to Central Institute for the Deaf and by Special Fellowship awards NS 1992 and NS 2052 from the National Institute of Neurological Diseases and Stroke to Dr Templer and to Dr Benitez.

REFERENCES

Huggins, W. H. and Licklider, J. C. R. (1951). Place mechanisms of auditory frequency analysis. *J. acoust. Soc. Am.*, **23**, 290–299.

Tasaki, I., Davis, H. and Legouix, J.-P. (1952). The space-time pattern of the cochlear microphonics (guinea pig), as recorded by differential electrodes. *J. acoust. Soc. Am.*, **24**, 502–519.

Teas, D. C., Eldredge, D. H. and Davis, H. (1962). Cochlear responses to acoustic transients: An interpretation of whole-nerve action potentials. *J. acoust. Soc. Am.*, **34**, 1438–1459.

Von Békésy, G. (1951). Microphonics produced by touching the cochlear partition with a vibrating electrode. *J. acoust. Soc. Am.*, **23**, 29–35.

Anatomical and Physiological Correlates of Threshold Shifts in the Chinchilla after Exposure to Noise

D. H. ELDREDGE

Central Institute for the Deaf, St Louis, Missouri, U.S.A.

INTRODUCTION

The list of variables related to hearing and to noise exposure that are under study in our laboratories is long. The list includes temporary and permanent shifts of behavioral auditory thresholds, temporary and permanent changes in the cochlear microphonic (CM) and whole-nerve action potential (AP), loss of hair cells and other measures of injury to the organ of Corti, and the characteristics of the noises that produced these changes. The matrix of relations between all pairs of the above variables is very large. For example, it is of great interest to know the relations between repeated episodes of temporary threshold shifts and the development of permanent threshold shifts, the anatomical losses associated with particular permanent threshold shifts, and so on.

During the past few years we have been developing methods and conducting studies that will help us to learn many of the important relations among the variables cited above. Miller (1970) has reported a method of instrumental avoidance conditioning that may be used to measure the thresholds of audibility for pure tones in the chinchilla. The normal thresholds for chinchilla are very similar to those for man in the low- and mid-frequency ranges and are about 30 dB to 40 dB more sensitive than man at 20 kHz. The cochlea of chinchilla protrudes in the auditory bulla with three turns that are accessible to differential electrodes. Thus we chose the chinchilla as an experimental animal because it was easily conditioned, had an auditory sensitivity similar to that of man, and had a cochlea that could be studied with our standard physiological methods.

METHODS

Behavioral Thresholds

Before an animal is trained, his left cochlea is surgically destroyed so that behaviorally-measured thresholds can be unambiguously associated with the right ear. This operation is done under general anesthesia with sterile procedures. After recovery from the surgery, the chinchilla is trained to move from one side to the other of an electrified double-grille cage to avoid electric shock when a tone is presented. A buzzer attached to and capable of vibrating the cage is paired with the shock and soon assumes most of the aversive properties of the shock. Then the less stressful buzzer is always used when testing near threshold. The psychophysical procedure used to obtain threshold at each frequency is an abbreviated or modified method of limits. To maintain good control over behavior each experimental session must be short. For this reason threshold reliability is established by averaging across several sessions rather than by averaging several determinations within a session.

Cochlear Microphonics

The measurement of physiological potentials is done under general anesthesia. Through a ventral surgical approach the auditory bulla is opened to expose the bony cochlea. Following the method of Tasaki et al. (1952) differential electrodes are inserted across each of the three cochlear turns. The acoustic system is a dynamic ear-phone sealed to the ear canal. CM outputs as a function of sound pressure level are measured at 200 Hz, 500 Hz and 1,000 Hz at the third, second and first turns respectively. The AP responses are also measured with the electrodes in the first turn. By taking the average voltages at these electrodes with respect to a remote reference on the neck wound, CM is greatly diminished and AP remains at its full voltage. The signal most commonly used is a wide-band click and the peak voltage of the N_1 is measured as a function of the click level.

Action Potentials

The wide-band click is the same as that depicted in the film, "Electrical Traveling Waves in the Chinchilla Cochlea" (Eldredge et al., 1973a). This click would appear to excite the major portion of the basilar membrane. Some additional refinement of the measures of AP responses was achieved by observing the masked and the residual N_1 responses to this click in appropriate bands of noise. The principles are the same as those described by Teas et al. (1962) but the averaging and the subtraction of traces is done with a LINC computer instead of hand-measured comparisons of multiply-exposed photographs. Briefly, the steps are as follows. At each click level there is some minimum wide-band noise level that will completely mask or disrupt the AP response. The electrical waveform for this noise is passed through a 6 kHz high-pass filter and mixed with the electrical square wave used to produce the click. The AP response with the noise present is subtracted from the AP response without the noise in order to know that part of the response that is not present and considered to be masked by the noise. This procedure is repeated with the high-pass filter set to 4 kHz, to 2 kHz, and to 1 kHz and the incremental loss of AP with each extension of the bandwidth of the noise to lower frequencies is similarly measured. If desired, separate input-output functions can be plotted for the AP masked by each incremental change in noise bandwith.

Histology

The cochleas were prepared for microscopic evaluation of injuries by either of two methods. The earlier, more classical method (Covell, 1953) employed intravital perfusion with saline followed by Heidenhain's susa. After decalcification in 3 per cent nitric acid and embedding in celloidin, 14 μm serial sections were cut parallel to the axis of the modiolus and every fifth section mounted and stained with hematoxylin and eosin. The injuries at each sample of the organ of Corti on these sections were evaluated under the microscope and plotted on a cochlear reconstruction.

A second method developed by Bohne (1972) grew out of methods reported earlier by Spoendlin (1966) and Kirchner (1968). After peri-lymphatic perfusion with osmic acid and dehydration in alcohols, the undissected cochlear portion of the temporal bone is infiltrated with the araldite plastic. The polymerized araldite provides excellent mech-anical support for the membranous labyrinth while the bony labyrinth is cut away with small steel picks and razor blades. Exposed segments of the membranous labyrinth are cut away from the modiolus and re-embedded in a flat block or wafer of araldite with the basilar membrane lying as close as possible to one surface. The organ of Corti may then be viewed as a flat preparation with a phase contrast microscope by focusing through the basilar membrane to the reticular lamina. Recon-struction of cochlear injuries is straightforward because the entire organ of Corti may be viewed from end to end. At areas of particular interest the araldite block may be cut perpendicular to the basilar membrane to obtain the more usual radial sections of the organ of Corti.

SECTION I

Exposure to Broad-band Noise for 3–4 Hours

The first examples of the kinds of experiments described above are taken from a larger study by J. D. Miller and D. H. Eldredge that is not yet complete. Four monaural chinchillas were exposed for 220 min in a diffuse sound field to broadband noise (250 Hz to 10 kHz) with an overall sound pressure level of 108 dB. One day after the exposure the behavioral thresholds were shifted by 60 dB to more than 95 dB at representative frequencies. A few weeks after the exposure threshold sensitivity improved considerably. By the end of three months the residual shifts in auditory thresholds appeared to be permanent. For frequencies above 1,400 Hz the permanent threshold shifts were about 60 dB in all four animals. Three animals showed permanent shifts of only 3–10 dB for frequencies below 1,000 Hz while the fourth showed an average shift of 25 dB for these frequencies.

Cochlear microphonics were measured differentially in each of the three cochlear turns. The losses of sensitivity were more than 60 dB in the basal turn, 30–60 dB in the second turn, and 15–50 dB in the third turn. The losses of maximum CM voltage were more than 30 dB, 25–30 dB, and 10–20 dB respectively. The whole-nerve AP in response to clicks contained no component that could be masked by high-frequency noise and showed the latencies logically associated with neural responses arising in the apical portions of the cochlea. In each instance less voltage was recorded from the ear of the one animal who had shown the greater threshold shifts for low frequencies.

The organ of Corti was completely absent in portions of the first turn of each ear. Through the basal 8–10 mm of the basilar membrane all outer hair cells were missing or clearly abnormal. Inner hair cells were still present in the area extending 1–2 mm from the round window and in the upper portions of the first turn. The organ of Corti was present in the second turns but showed frequent missing, defective, and detached hair cells. In the third turn the organ of Corti more nearly approached normal appearance. Corresponding losses of neurons were observed at different levels of the spiral ganglion.

Exposure to Octave-band Noise for 3–4 Hours

Von Bismarck (1967) measured on chinchillas the ratios of sound pressures at the tympanic membrane to those in the field. At frequencies up to about 1,000 Hz these ratios were never more than a few decibels. However, the presence of the head and pinna and the resonances of the outer canal produced ratios of about 20 dB in the range of frequencies from about 2 kHz to about 4 kHz. For this reason one might expect exposures to noise with acoustic energy in this band of frequencies to be more injurious than when the energy is at other frequencies. One of two chinchillas who had been exposed to a band of noise from 2–4 kHz at 101 dB SPL for 216 min presented interesting relations among noise exposure, permanent behavioral threshold shift, cochlear potentials and cochlear injury. The spectrum level for this band was the same as for the exposure to wide-band noise but the overall level was 7 dB less.

One day after exposure the behavioral thresholds were normal at 500 Hz and below, and shifted by 50–75 dB for frequencies above 2,000 Hz. Three months later the behavioral thresholds were normal and at pre-exposure levels except for a permanent shift of 25 dB at 2,000 Hz. The CM responses were normal in the first and third turns but about 25 per cent (-12 dB) of normal values in the second turn. The AP responses were significantly lower than normal and the masked responses showed unusual relations. One component was masked by frequencies above 6 kHz in a nearly normal manner, but as noise at lower frequencies was added first to 4 kHz, then to 2 kHz, very little more masking occurred. Finally the addition of frequencies below 2 kHz completed the masking in a more usual way.

The cochlear reconstruction showed that all outer hair cells were absent for a distance of about 1 mm centered in an area 7 mm from the stapes end of the basilar membrane. In this area many, but not all, Deiters' cells were also absent, but the tunnel of Corti and the inner hair cells were in normal positions. For about 0·5 mm at either end of the lesion there may have been other outer hair cells that had been displaced from their normal positions but were still present. The sections were on chords rather than radii in these areas so that precise relations were difficult to interpret. In any event, this injury was clearly not so severe as for the wide-band noise with the same spectrum level but a higher overall level.

Prolonged Exposures to Octave-band Noise

The details of a third exposure to noise are being reported separately (Miller *et al.*, 1971) because the results lead directly to several other studies. From the measurements of von Bismarck (1967) cited above one would predict that for low frequencies either higher sound pressures in the field or very much longer durations of exposure would be necessary to injure the ear. Two chinchillas were exposed continuously for seven days to an octave band of noise from 300–600 Hz at 100 dB SPL. For this exposure the spectrum level was 7 dB above that for the exposure to the wide-band noise even though the overall level was 8 dB less. The sensitivity of the behavioral auditory thresholds continued to decrease for 24–48 hours and then stabilized asymptotically at new levels during the remainder of the exposure. Those frequencies within and just above the band of noise showed the largest thresholds shifts. These asymptotic levels were about 55 dB above corresponding normal thresholds.

Three months later the behavioral thresholds had returned to within 5 dB of their normal, pre-exposure levels at most frequencies and within 10 dB at all others. Although the residual differences fell within the standard error of the means for these techniques, the trends of the deviations suggested permanent losses of sensitivity of about 5 dB at some of the appropriate low frequencies. These were accompanied by small, but significant losses of sensitivity in CM and AP. In the second and third cochlear turns there was scattered loss of outer hair cells. These losses did not form continuous lesions but the cells were clearly missing even on the samples provided when using only every fifth section.

DISCUSSION

The three examples described above invite several broad conclusions concerning possible relations among exposures to noise, auditory thresholds, cochlear potentials and cochlear injury. The word "possible" is used deliberately because not all arguments from the observations are symmetrical. For example, it seems certain that an absent hair cell cannot contribute to hearing or to cochlear potentials. However, we do not know that all or any hair cells remaining in or near areas of injury to the organ of Corti can or do function normally. In the first example when there was large, complete loss of the organ of Corti in the first turn and loss of all outer hair cells from this area of total loss to the round window, a few remaining inner hair cells sufficed to detect high-frequency tones at levels 60 dB above normal thresholds. Under more favorable circumstances these same inner hair cells might be more sensitive than this indication. In the second example a permanent behavioral threshold shift of only 25 dB at a single frequency reflected a total loss of outer hair cells for a distance of 1 mm at an appropriate place. The cells responsible for hearing at the elevated threshold could have been the remaining inner hair cells or the traveling wave pattern could have spread to intact organ of Corti in adjacent areas. The third example showed that a diffuse scattered loss of hair cells in the second and third turns was accompanied by little (5 dB) or no loss of sensitivity for the behavioral threshold responses to pure tones.

SECTION II

Carder and Miller (1972) explored more thoroughly several of the relations indicated in Section I when the temporary shifts in behavioral auditory thresholds reached asymptotic values during very long exposures to noise. They exposed chinchillas to an octave band of noise centered at 500 Hz continuously for periods ranging from 2 to 21 days. Behavioral thresholds at 715 Hz were observed to grow less sensitive with continued exposure for 24 hours and then to stabilize at an asymptotic value. When the octave band values were 75, 85, 95, and 105 dB SPL the shifts in behavioral threshold were about 17, 31, 49, and 63 dB respectively. Recovery to normal thresholds required 2 to 7 days with the larger threshold shifts requiring the longer times. However, recoveries to normal from exposures at 85 dB SPL for 2, 7, and 21 days were identical. For this reason it was inferred that each asymptotic condition represented a state of equilibrium. This state presented an opportunity to explore some of the physiological correlates of temporary threshold shifts.

Similar asymptotic temporary shifts of auditory thresholds in one man were reported by Mills *et al.* (1970). In man the asymptote appeared to be reached in only 8–12 hours, but recovery was similarly slow requiring two days to recover from a shift of only 10·5 dB in sensitivity. Mosko *et al.* (1970) confirms the asymptote in man.

Benitez *et al.* (1971) measured the changes in cochlear potentials following exposures to the octave band of noise centered at 500 Hz with an SPL of 95 dB for two or three days. The changes that corresponded most closely to the behavioral threshold shifts were the changes in sensitivity of the CM responses in the three cochlear turns as these were measured 5, 24, and 48 hours after the ends of the exposures. Rather surprisingly the changes in sensitivity for the AP responses to the wide-band click greatly exceeded the changes in behavioral thresholds. No AP responses could be measured at levels 90 dB above normal thresholds four to six hours after the end of exposure. However, average evoked responses similar to those measured by Henderson *et al.* (1969) were observed in response to the wide-band click only 30 min after the end of exposures. The change in threshold for these evoked responses of 40–50 dB was about the same as the change in behavioral thresholds and in the sensitivity for CM.

DISCUSSION

Studies such as the ones cited above suggest that on continued long exposure to noise the auditory system loses sensitivity until some kind of state of equilibrium is reached. We assume that the processes that diminish sensitivity are then just equal and opposite to those that restore sensitivity. In any event the pure tone thresholds become stable. In physiological terms the changes in sensitivity for CM can account for the total loss of sensitivity that is observed behaviorally. There is no need to adduce additional losses more centrally in the auditory system.

However, the whole-nerve AP responses to clicks and to tonal onsets show greater losses in sensitivity and are poor indices of the behavioral deficits. Tentatively we must postulate that there is a combination of loss of sensitivity and loss of synchrony in order to account for the loss of AP voltage. There must be some appropriate activity in the auditory nerve because an averaged evoked response that appears to arise in the brain stem at the level of the inferior colliculi (Rothenberg and Davis, 1967; Henderson et al., 1969) can be observed at levels consistent with the behavioral thresholds.

SECTION III

Eldredge et al. (1973b) described some anatomical, behavioral and physiological observations on chinchillas after a relatively long exposure to noise. Four monaural chinchillas were exposed continuously for 24 days to an octave band of noise centered at 4 kHz. The total exposure was divided into four periods of six days each during which the band levels were 57 dB, 65 dB, 72 dB and 80 dB in that order (Mills et al., 1970). For each level of exposure the behavioral thresholds shifted to a new asymptotic loss of sensitivity. During the exposure at 80 dB the mean threshold shift for the group reached an asymptote at 54 dB for 5·7 kHz, the frequency with the greatest threshold shift. This group of animals attracted our attention because their behavioral thresholds had not returned to normal pre-exposure hearing levels 14 days after the termination of the exposure. Other chinchillas with similar temporary threshold shifts had completely recovered in three to six days.

Cochlear Pathology

The ear from each chinchilla was examined in detail using the method of araldite-embedded flat preparations. All ears showed injuries to the organ of Corti in a region of the first turn appropriate to frequencies around 4 kHz. The numbers of missing outer hair cells were approximately 20, 50, 70 and 290 in each of the four ears. In the ear with the least injury there was only one injured pillar cell and in the ear with the most injury there were several places with loss of all hair and pillar cells. These latter lesions were scattered through a distance of about one millimeter with the longest single lesion being only about one-tenth millimeter.

Behavioral Auditory Thresholds

Behavioral thresholds were measured repeatedly during the period 84–98 days after the termination of the exposure and mean audiograms were plotted for each ear. Except at 16 kHz no threshold differed by more than 8 dB from the mean, normal values reported by Miller (1970).

Both before and after exposure the hearing levels at 16 kHz were about 15 dB less sensitive than the mean, normal values. None of the differences from normal or between pre-exposure and post-exposure hearing levels was significant at any frequency for any ear. Nor were there any significant differences between the hearing levels for the ears with the least and with the most injury.

Cochlear Potentials

The normal differential CM voltage is considered to be contributed by a length of the organ of Corti that lies within one millimeter either side of the electrodes. This model for CM also implies that if it were possible to remove all of the hair cell sources of CM over this one millimeter on either side of the electrodes without changing other electrical properties or injuring other hair cells, then CM should be reduced by only 6 dB at each input sound pressure level. The injuries to the organ of Corti were all small and discontinuous relative to the above hypothesized loss. Accordingly one might expect for the ear with 290 missing outer hair cells a loss of less than 6 dB. For the ears with smaller injuries the CM responses should be nearly normal. The input-output function for the ear with about 50 missing outer hair cells was within one standard deviation below the normal mean values, but the three other ears produced voltages that were two to four standard deviations below the normal means. For these ears the loss of maximum CM voltage was only 2 dB, but it was accompanied by losses of sensitivity of 6–12 dB. We do not know why the observed losses in sensitivity were greater than the hypothesized losses. The input-output functions for the least and most injured ears were almost identical. Thus measures of CM were not sensitive to these differences in anatomical injury.

The best indices for the relatively small cochlear injuries proved to be the whole-nerve AP and the component masked by the 6-kHz high-pass noise. The N_1 peak voltage as a function of click level was clearly normal for the ear with only about 20 missing outer hair cells. The N_1 component masked by the 6-kHz noise also grew normally for this ear. For the ears with about 50 and with about 70 missing outer hair cells N_1 values were systematically about one and two standard deviations respectively below mean normal values. The N_1 voltages were even smaller for the ear with about 290 missing outer hair cells. The maximum N_1 peak voltage reached only 30 per cent of normal and the N_1 component masked by the 6-kHz high-pass noise reached only 25 per cent of normal.

Even though the N_1 peak voltages proved to be a good index of injury, the relations do not appear to be consistent with quantitative measures of injury. In the most injured ear at least 70 per cent of hair cells remained in the 3-mm length that constituted the most affected area, yet AP voltages were reduced to 30 per cent of normal or less. Since we cannot account for the loss of N_1 voltage by quantitative measures of anatomical injury, we must assume that the reduced voltages represent loss of synchrony as well as loss of active units.

CONCLUDING REMARKS

Comprehensive quantitative statements about the relations between and among the dimensions cited in the Introduction are premature. However, we appear to have some indications concerning the nature of some key relations. For example, it is becoming clear that we can find small cochlear injuries in the absence of permanent behavioral threshold shifts. Complete absence of outer hair cells for a distance of about a millimeter may be reflected by a threshold shift of only 20 dB. Yet when there is complete absence of organ of Corti for several millimeters in the middle of the basal turn, a relatively few inner hair cells remaining near the round window may serve to detect high-frequency tones at levels 60 dB above the normal thresholds.

The existence of an asymptotic state of temporary threshold shift is interesting from several points of view. First, those longer exposures at lower levels more closely approximate industrial exposures to noise. In this regard the few measures we have for man (Mills *et al.*, 1970) suggest that in man the asymptote is reached in about 8–12 hours, or about a working day. Recovery to normal thresholds is always slower than one might expect from previous laboratory experiments employing shorter exposures and may require at least two days for either man or chinchilla. In chinchilla exposures to levels of noise that produce asymptotic shifts in behavioral thresholds of 50 dB or more have repeatedly produced small, but definite, cochlear injuries. Such injuries may be, but are not always, associated with delayed recovery to normal behavioral thresholds.

We have looked at some of the relations of three physiological responses (CM, whole-nerve AP, and averaged auditory evoked response) to anatomical injury and to both temporary and permanent shifts of behavioral auditory thresholds. The synchronized AP responses appeared to be the most sensitive index of injury and were significantly diminished when CM responses were less significantly diminished and when behavioral thresholds were normal. When behavioral thresholds, either permanent or temporary, were shifted by 20 dB to about 55 dB, there were corresponding and roughly equivalent changes in sensitivity for the CM responses and often greater losses in sensitivity for the AP responses. When the behavioral thresholds were shifted by 60 dB or more, CM responses could not always be obtained. We do not yet have enough data to support basic statements about the normal and pathological relations between CM and AP. For the present we observe that the whole-nerve AP is the most sensitive index for small injuries to the cochlea. As the injuries become larger the AP is so severely affected that it does not seem possible to use it to discriminate between varying degrees of moderate to severe injury. Here the CM seems to be correlated more closely with the degree of injury. With different methods for measuring AP or with different models for CM it may be possible to interpret changes in these potentials over a wider dynamic range of injury or threshold shift. Now, the averaged auditory evoked responses appear to be the measure that relates quantatitively to behavioral thresholds over the widest dynamic range.

ACKNOWLEDGEMENTS

The work for this paper was supported by Research Grant NS 03856, from the National Institute of Neurological Diseases to the Central Institute for the Deaf.

REFERENCES

Benitez, L. D., Eldredge, D. H. and Templer, J. W. (1971). Electrophysiological correlates of behavioral temporary threshold shifts in chinchilla. *J. acoust. Soc. Am.*, **49**, 121(A).

Bismarck, von G. (1967). The Sound Pressure Transformation Function from Free-Field to the Eardrum of Chinchilla. M.S. thesis. MIT, Cambridge, Mass.

Bohne, B. A. (1972). Location of small cochlear lesions by phase contrast microscopy prior to thin sectioning. *Laryngoscope*. (In press.)

Carder, H. M. and Miller, J. D. (1972). Temporary threshold shifts produced by noise exposures of long duration. *Trans. Am. Acad. Ophthalmol. Otolaryngol,,* **75**, 1346–1352.

Covell, W. P. (1953). Histologic changes in the organ of Corti with intense sound. *J. comp. Neur.*, **99**, 43–60.

Eldredge, D. H., Benitez, L. D. and Templer, J. W. (1973a). Film: Electrical traveling waves in the chinchilla cochlea. *Sound*. (In press.)

Eldredge, D. H., Mills, J. H. and Bohne, B. A. (1973b). Anatomical, behavioral, and electrophysiological observations on chinchillas after long exposure to noise. To be published in the proceedings of *International Symposium on Otophysiology*, Univ. of Michigan Medical Center, 20–22 May 1971.

Henderson, D., Onishi, S., Eldredge, D. H. and Davis, H. (1969). A comparison of chinchilla auditory evoked response and behavioral response thresholds. *Percept. Psychophys.* **5**, 41–45.

Kirchner, F. R. (1968). Intralabyrinthine perfusion. *Laryngoscope*, **78**, 2049–2118.

Miller, J. D. (1970). Audibility curve of the chinchilla. *J. acoust. Soc. Am.*, **48**, 513–523.

Miller, J. D., Rothenberg, S. J. and Eldredge, D. H. (1971). Preliminary observations on the effects of exposure to noise for seven days on the hearing and inner ear of the chinchilla. *J. acoust. Soc. Am.*, **50**, 1199–1203.

Mills, J. H. (1971). Temporary threshold shifts produced by prolonged exposure to high-frequency noise. *J. acoust. Soc. Am.*, **49**, 92(A).

Mills, J. H., Gengel, R. W., Watson, C. S. and Miller, J. D. (1970). Temporary changes of the auditory system due to exposure to noise for one or two days. *J. acoust. Soc. Am.*, **48**, 524–530.

Mosko, J. D., Fletcher, J. L. and Luz, G. A. (1970). "Growth and Recovery of Temporary Threshold Shifts Following Extended Exposure to High-Level, Continuous Noise". U.S. AMRL Rept. 911, Fort Knox, Ky. 9 pp.

Rothenberg, S. and Davis, H. (1967). Auditory evoked response in chinchilla: Application to animal audiometry. *Percept. Psychophys.*, **2**, 443–447.

Spoendlin, H. (1966). "The Organization of the Cochlear Receptor". S. Karger, Basel, Switzerland.

Tasaki, I., Davis, H. and Legouix, J.-P. (1952). The space-time patterns of the cochlear microphonics (guinea pig), as recorded by differential electrodes. *J. acoust. Soc. Am.*, **24**, 502–519.

Teas, D. C., Eldredge, D. H. and Davis, H. (1962). Cochlear responses to acoustic transients: An interpretation of whole-nerve action potentials. *J. acoust. Soc. Am.*, **34**, 1438–1459.

Foetal Audiometry in Relation to the Developing Foetal Nervous System

J. BENCH

*Audiology Research Unit, Royal Berkshire Hospital,
Reading, England*

Recently there has been a large number of rather brief publications by workers in the fields of audiology, infant neurology, obstetrics and otology who have attempted to measure human foetal response to acoustic stimuli. A careful review indicates to me that in much of this work important controls have been omitted, and that there has been little attempt to relate empirical endeavours to what is known of the developing foetal nervous system. I propose in this paper to take a rather extreme position in which I shall try to state a case for claiming that the foetus is rather *un*responsive to sensory stimulation. I do not necessarily feel that this position is the "right" one, but if a reasonable case can be made for claiming that the foetus is relatively *in*sensitive to, or even *un*responsive to, auditory and other stimuli, we must regard claims for successful measure of foetal response to sound with caution.

I propose firstly to outline briefly some current techniques in what, for want of a better term, I call foetal audiometry; secondly to describe briefly some controls which seem important; and thirdly to discuss at somewhat greater length the relation of such work to some aspects of the foetal nervous system.

TECHNIQUES FOR GENERATING STIMULI AND ASSESSING RESPONSE

The most viable approach is probably to stimulate the foetus with audio-frequency signals via a vibrator mechanically coupled to the maternal abdomen, and to monitor heart rate changes, as pioneered by Sontag (1936, 1944), and continued by Murphy and Smyth (1962), Johansson *et al.* (1964) and Bench *et al.* (1970). Some workers have attempted to use the foetal EEG, monitored via maternal abdominal

I

electrodes, as their dependent variable. I have attempted to use this technique myself, but found it difficult and rather unreliable. The foetal EEG signals were small, and difficult to extract from physiological noise.

CONTROLS

It is convenient to break down the discussion of controls by considering them under two headings: procedural and statistical. In *procedural controls*, we must consider:

(*a*) preventing the mother from hearing the foetal stimulus, and influencing the foetus by a secondary (e.g. humoral) stimulation; (*b*) pre-exposure of the mother to experimental methods to allay anxiety, which may affect the foetus as in (*a*); (*c*) avoiding uterine contractions or taking their effects on foetal physiology into account; (*d*) allowing for geometrical factors which change with advancing pregnancy, and with the posture of the mother during investigations; and (*e*) obtaining an efficient transducer coupling for audio frequency signals, thus ensuring that sufficient energy reaches the foetal ear.

In *statistical controls*, we must consider:

(*a*) the spontaneous regression of foetal activity to some mean or intermediate value; and (*b*) assessing any effects occasioned by the Law of Initial Value (Wilder, 1957).

A study of the literature on stimulation through the maternal abdominal wall of the surgically undisturbed foetus, particularly in work on the human foetus for which responses to vibratory stimuli were claimed, indicates that in much of the early work important controls were missing. Thus although non-stimulus control trials had been included by Sontag and co-workers (1936, 1944), the control of preventing the mother from hearing sounds played to the foetus, and herself influencing foetal activity via e.g. hormones, was omitted. This omission seems particularly important, since some of Sontag's results suggest a long foetal response latency, which might be due to humoral stimulation from the mother. In other work (Murphy and Smyth, 1962), which Bench and Vass (1970) failed to replicate, the mother was prevented from hearing the foetal stimulus, but no non-stimulus control periods were employed.

In more recent work on audio-frequency stimulation of the human foetus, Johansson *et al.* (1964), Bench and Mittler (1967) and Smyth and Bench (1967), prevented the mother from hearing the foetal stimulus and included non-stimulus control periods. These results offer more convincing support for the responsivity of surgically undisturbed foetuses to auditory stimulation. However, in these cases, non-stimulus control periods were taken from the period immediately before the stimulus trials. A better control would have been to make stimulus and non-stimulus equivalent in time.

THE RELATION OF FOETAL AUDIOMETRY TO ASPECTS OF THE FOETAL NERVOUS SYSTEM

When the literature on empirical tests of sensory function in the foetus is examined, it seems at first impression as though there is overwhelming evidence for the validity of foetal response to stimulation in a number of sensory modalities (see Carmichael's review, 1951). Nevertheless, when this evidence is examined more closely, it is apparent that much of the work has been performed on the exteriorized or partially exteriorized animal foetus, and not on the foetus in utero with the membranes, etc., intact.

Barcroft and Barron (1937) exteriorized sheep foetuses and tapped them on the snout with a glass rod. They found that startles elicited by such tapping early in pregnancy disappeared at a later stage. There is thus some direct evidence to suggest that parts at least of nervous function in even the exteriorized sheep foetus are under some kind of inhibition or depression* which develops during gestation. It may be that the development of this inhibition is linked in time with the anatomical development of some sensory pathways, which thus do not have an opportunity to function fully in utero. Since exteriorization of the foetus may break the inhibition, demonstrations of sensory function in the exteriorized foetus do not necessarily prove that the foetus undergoes similar experiences in the undisturbed uterus.

As another example of such depression, aspects of respiratory and crying activity seem to be checked until birth in the human foetus (although the appropriate nervous centres are fully developed at birth) since otherwise the foetus could fill his lungs with amniotic liquor, and "drown from the inside" at birth with the onset of air respiration. The regular movements of the foetal chest noted by Ahlfeld (1890) and which may be related to actions which will later be necessary in breathing do not normally lead to inspiration of the amniotic fluid (Windle, 1941). Evidence of yet another kind for this depression comes from the results of Riesen (1947) in experiments on chimpanzees reared in darkness. Riesen's results, which showed that deprivation of light after birth led to retarded development of visually mediated behaviour, seem to suggest that the chimpanzee's visual nervous system is not functioning until birth—otherwise they are difficult to interpret. Wedenberg *et al.* (1964),

---

* The terms "inhibition" and "depression" are used here in a general sense, and not in a specific neurological or psychological sense.

have considered this point briefly, with regard to auditory and visual stimulation of the human foetus:

> Through this (sound) stimulation (of the human foetus) the formation of the nucleo-protein fraction in ganglion cochleare starts. Contrary to this, the vision can never be stimulated before birth. The newborn in the first day of life to a great extent lacks the nucleo-protein fraction in ganglion ciliare and as a consequence has very little, if any, capacity to see in the first days.

If this statement is reliable then the depression discussed above is perhaps not complete, but applies only to parts of the foetal nervous system.

I realize, of course, that response inhibition on the one hand and depression or inhibition of sensory mechanisms on the other are two separate issues. To fail to demonstrate adequately a response to stimulation is not necessarily to demonstrate a lack of sensory experience, since it may be only the response which is inhibited, and not the sensory input. Nevertheless, the fact that some kind of inhibition is thought to occur in both the animal and human foetal nervous system makes it necessary, in the absence of evidence resolving the issue of stimulus/response inhibition, to treat reports of the sensory capacities of the foetus with caution.

REFERENCES

Ahlfeld, J. F. (1890). *In* Beitrage zur Physiologie. Festschrift zu Care Ludwig zu seinem 70. Gebutstage gewidmet von seinen Schulern. Vogel, Leipzig, pp. 1–32.

Barcroft, T. and Barron, D. H. (1937). Movements in midfoetal life in the sheep embryo. *J. Physiol.*, **91**, 329–351.

Bench, R. J. and Mittler, P. J. (1967). Changes of heart rate in response to auditory stimulation in the human foetus, *Abstr. Bull. Brit. Psychol. Soc.*, **20**, 14A.

Bench, R. J. and Vass, A. (1970). Fetal audiometry, *Lancet*, **1**, 91–92.

Bench, R. J., Anderson, J. H. and Hoare, M. (1970). Measurement System for Fetal Audiometry, *J. acoust. Soc. Am.*, **47**, 1602–1606.

Carmichael, L. (1951). *In* "Handbook of Experimental Psychology" (S. S. Stevens, ed.), pp. 281–303.

Johansson, B., Wedenberg, E. and Westin, B. (1964). Measurement of tone response by the human foetus, *Acta Otolaryng.*, **57**, 188–192.

Murphy, K. P. and Smyth, C. N. (1962). Response of fetus to auditory stimulation, *Lancet*, **1**, 972–973.

Riesen, A. H. (1947). The development of visual perception in man and chimpanzee, *Science*, **106**, 107–108.

Smyth, C. N. and Bench, R. J. (1967). Fetal response to audiogenic stimulation as an indication of neurological function, *Digest 7th Int. Conf. Med. Biol. Engng.*, 137–139.

Sontag, L. W. (1936). Changes in the rate of human fetal heart in response to vibratory stimuli, *Am. J. Dis. Child.*, **51**. 538–589.

Sontag, L. W. (1944). Differences in modifiability of fetal behavior and physiology, *Psychosom. Med.*, **6**, 151–154.

Wedenberg, E., Johansson, B. and Westin, B. (1964). Measurement of tone response by the human foetus. *In* "Neonate Hearing". Int. Conf. in Copenhagen.

Wilder, J. (1957). The Law of Initial Value in neurology and psychiatry: facts and problems. *J. Nerv. Ment. Dis.*, **125**, 73–86.

Windle, W. F. (1941). Physiology and anatomy of the respiratory system in the foetus and newborn infant, *J. Paediat.*, **19**, 437–444.

The Callier Hearing and Speech Center, Dallas, Texas

A. GLORIG

The Callier Hearing and Speech Center, Dallas, Texas, U.S.A.

PURPOSE AND NEED

The Callier Hearing and Speech Center serves a community of two and one-half million people and is the only agency in this community that is devoted primarily to problems of human communication. When the population projection of individuals having problems in human communication is based on the total population of Callier's service area, the communication-impaired population (including those with hearing and speech problems) would be approximately 175,000 as a conservative estimate. The very size of the problem places a heavy responsibility on the Callier Center.

During 1967, the Callier Hearing and Speech Center provided broad service in the communications disorders field for 8,700 persons.

The Callier Center moved to its new facilities on 26 July 1968. With the increase in space, there has been an increase in services to the point that it is now projected that patients being served by the Center will reach at least 25,000 for the year 1972. The rapid rise in requests for patient services suggests that the present staff will be unable to handle adequately the amount of services that will be needed.

The Callier Hearing and Speech Center's concept of community service involves the provision of needed services throughout the community, even when the patient cannot come to the Center. At present, a city-wide program of aphasia therapy is underway, with the need for speech therapy services for patients in nursing homes and at home growing weekly.

The case load in audiology is growing much more rapidly than was anticipated when the move to the new facilities was made. Two major problems have arisen in this regard: Firstly, the need for almost-immediate evaluations on patients referred by otologists when tests for localization of neurosensory lesions are matters of urgency; and secondly, the waiting time before less urgent evaluations can be scheduled. The Callier Hearing and Speech Center has attempted to establish no longer than two weeks between referral and appointment. This is no longer possible with the present staff. In addition, audiologists are being requested to work with more and more hearing-aid users in rehabilitative services such as auditory training, speech reading, and speech improvement. A number of these referrals are coming from hearing-aid dealers, which is unique throughout most of the nation but so highly desirable that all efforts are being made to provide the requested services.

The Callier Center has space for eight complete testing suites for conducting complete evaluations of hearing difficulties.

Another aspect of the Callier service involves the early identification and diagnosis of infants with hearing problems. Although the Center now has a program of infant testing as soon as the child is permitted to come to the Center, it is obvious that many of the "high risk category" children are not tested at an early age and, therefore, may be severely delayed in language and speech development. One of the more important projections of service is the initiation of an infant screening program at the earliest possible date. The increase in infant referrals to the Center for further testing will necessitate an increase in the audiological staff.

Although we accept patients from a few weeks old to senior citizens, 70 per cent of our patient load is under 16 years of age. Services are provided on a fee basis, which is adjusted to the individual's ability to pay. All patients whose income is under $8,000 annually are interviewed by our social service department and are charged according to ability to pay. A large percentage of our patient load is in a low income bracket; however, the services are the same for all. The Callier Center maintains a high professional level of service for all patients regardless of ability to pay. Although costly, the Callier Hearing and Speech Center functions as a community center and believes strongly that this is our obligation.

Since moving to our new facilities, our patient load has increased significantly, as previously outlined. We expect a still larger increase in the need for the services of the Center. To maintain a high quality of service to communications impaired individuals, we must have additional staff members qualified to carry out these needed services.

ORGANIZATION AND ADMINISTRATION

The Callier Hearing and Speech Center was organized in 1964 following a lengthy period of time devoted to a study of the needs of the community in which it was to be built. The original impetus for the Center came from the trust established under the will of Mrs Lena Callier. The final decisions concerning the use of this trust were made by a committee composed of civic-minded, influential citizens of the Dallas community. Before final decisions were made, studies were made by specialists including representatives of Health, Education and Welfare, the National Association of Hearing and Speech Agencies, and several appropriate consultants in the field of hearing and communications rehabilitation.

Three already-existing agencies in Dallas were merged into a cooperative program combining those services to which each had been previously devoted. These agencies were the Pilot School for the Deaf, the Dallas Speech and Hearing Center, and the Dallas Council for the Deaf. Expansion of services was planned along specific lines both to enlarge existing services as well as to add new service areas suggested by the studies made of community needs.

The Center is now organized to offer services related to all types of human communication disorders. The organizational structure of the Callier Center includes one Director, Aram Glorig, M.D., and four Associate Directors. The Center has three main service divisions, as follows.

1. Clinical Services Division.
    (a) Hearing, language and speech evaluations.
    (b) Programs of non-medical, non-surgical therapy for hearing, language and speech problems.
    (c) Otolaryngological evaluations.
    (d) Psychological evaluations.
    (e) Social service and counselling.
    (f) Adult deaf counselling and training.
    (g) Training program in cooperation with area universities (Southern Methodist University, Texas Woman's University, Southwestern Medical School, and North Texas State University).
2. Educational Division.
    (a) School for the deaf (primarily oral methods) (Age range: Infants, preschool, elementary school, 0–8 years) (9–21, associated with Dallas City School System).
    (b) Parent training.
        (Heaviest emphasis in infant and preschool areas.)
    (c) Training program in teacher training of educators of the deaf in cooperation with Texas Woman's University and Southern Methodist University.
3. Research Division.
    (a) Basic investigation of hearing and speech mechanisms.
    (b) Clinical investigations and applied research.

An organizational chart is shown as Fig. 1.

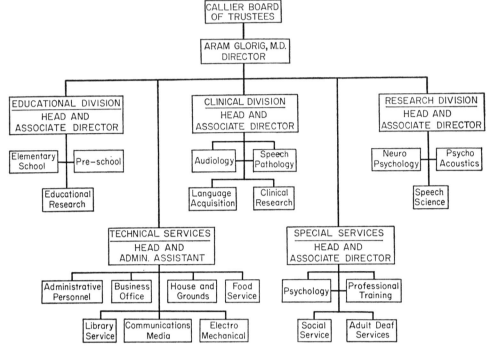

FIG. 1.

4. Special Services Division.
   (a) Provides supportive service for the clinical and educational divisions, including psychological, sociological and counselling. This division's principal purpose is to provide these services to the other divisions on a consultative basis.
5. Technical Services Section.

   This section provides all divisions with technical assistance including electrical, mechanical, audio visual and library service.

   The Center is completely wired for closed circuit television, which can be interfaced with community closed circuit systems for educational purposes. All divisions including administration have access to a self-contained computer system.

Two advisory committees have been appointed whose services are utilized in broad planning of service programs. An Administrative Committee composed of representatives of local service and educational agencies acts as an advisory group to the Director. A Scientific Advisory group is composed of individuals from various areas of the nation who are outstanding in their professional fields and who consult with the Director on professional matters pertinent to the service programs of the Center.

The Callier Hearing and Speech Center is affiliated with the Southwestern Medical School of the University of Texas located in Dallas; it is affiliated with Parkland Hospital and Children's Medical Center; it is affiliated with Southern Methodist University, Dallas; and with Texas Woman's University, Denton. The Director is on the staff of the Southwestern Medical School and staff members regularly lecture to medical students, interns and residents. Callier personnel work in the Division of Otolaryngology and the Department of Physical Medicine of the Southwestern Medical School and at Parkland Hospital. Callier personnel serve on special staffings at both Parkland Hospital and Children's Medical Center. Some are engaged in teaching assignments at Southern Methodist University and the Center serves as the primary area for graduate practicums in both audiology and speech pathology for students from area universities. Students enrolled in a teacher training program in deaf education at Texas Woman's University engage in practice teaching at the Educational Division of the Callier Center.

In addition to the professional affiliations listed above, the Center also provides services to:

1. Caruth Memorial Rehabilitation Center, a community center with both in-patient and out-patient programs. Callier personnel furnish all evaluation and therapy programs for those with human communication problems.
2. Department of Physical Medicine and Rehabilitation, St Paul's Hospital. Callier personnel serve as evaluators and consultants to patients during hospital tenure, as well as plan and carry out therapy afterward.
3. Department of Physical Medicine and Rehabilitation, Baylor Hospital. The same program is carried out in this facility as listed above.
4. Scottish Rite Hospital. Callier personnel serve as consultants in hearing and speech to this facility which is a state-wide hospital for crippled children.

In addition, the Callier Hearing and Speech Center works with the local school districts in the identification and evaluation of children with hearing problems and in cases of children with difficult diagnostic problems in language and speech. A special summer clinic has been held for four years to aid those students referred from school districts for special work during the summer school vacation. The need for enlargement of this program is obvious, since the clinic had to be limited last summer in part because of lack of adequate funding for the program.

Although a certain amount of community planning was done prior to the move to the new facilities, lack of space and personnel prevented the implementation of additional service programs. Now that the Callier Center is in new facilities with adequate space, a series of conferences with representatives from other community agencies have been scheduled for discussion of cooperative service programs. Inter-agency staffings have been planned and the first held, with expectations of a great expansion of such a program of cooperation between agencies handling mutual patient loads. Included in planning sessions and inter-agency staffings will be such community agencies as Dallas Services for Blind Children, Children's Development Center, Dallas Child Guidance Clinic, Family Guidance Center, etc.

Another type of community planning involves services to the adult deaf, and a program of adult education has already been initiated. Planning is underway for the use of the local educational television station for a wider coverage of such programs as well as planning for a course in sign language for those who wish to learn to communicate with the adult, non-oral deaf community. The Dallas community has an unusually large population of these individuals, and it is a growing number because of both employment and educational opportunities. Expansion of Callier's program in this area is considered an important contribution to community services.

PROGRAM OF SERVICES

The desired objectives to be met involve primarily an expansion of services already available so that the increase in patient load may be cared for without loss of quality of services; in fact, the addition of personnel to achieve these ends would be weighed carefully so that quality of services would be enhanced.

SPECIAL PROGRAMS

1. Deaf-Blind Program.

    The Center administrates a four-state program for deaf-blind children. Under this program, the Center operates a day school for preschool deaf-blind children. This program is used as a model for the eighteen deaf-blind schools conducted in the four state area.

2. Individualized Instruction Project.

This project is designed to study programmed learning techniques. The staff develops devices and material and sets up trials on matched groups to study their efficacy.

To summarize, community planning and cooperation will be continued in the areas of expansion of service programs, educational programs, and counselling programs for those with all types of communication problems.

An Index of Hearing Impairment derived from the Pure-Tone Audiogram

J. C. G. PEARSON, R. L. KELL*
and W. TAYLOR

*Department of Social and Occupational Medicine,
University of Dundee, Dundee, Scotland*

INTRODUCTION

Noise-induced hearing loss in female jute weavers in Dundee was studied retrospectively by Taylor *et al.* (1965) using pure-tone threshold audiometry. Considerable losses were found, especially at frequencies 2 kHz and above, when this population was compared with non-noise-exposed populations (Hinchcliffe, 1959; Taylor *et al.* 1967; Kell *et al.*, 1970).

A further study on female weavers in Dundee and district extended the investigation to include speech audiometry and a questionnaire concerning the social consequences of hearing loss (Kell *et al.*, 1971).

In social terms, the most important effect of hearing loss is difficulty in the understanding of speech. Consequently, the three audiometric frequencies in the centre of the band which is most important for the reception of speech, namely 0·5, 1 and 2 kHz, have been used empirically in an attempt to assess impairment from the pure-tone audiogram. Glorig (1959) proposed the use of the average hearing loss at these three frequencies for this assessment, and scales of impairment have been devised for occupational hearing loss in the U.S.A. (Davis and Kranz, 1964; Fox, 1965; Glorig, 1966). This "three average" method of assessment has been compared with answers to a hearing questionnaire to form a "hearing handicap scale" by High *et al.* (1964) using 50 subjects in the age range 21 to 72 years, who presented themselves with an unspecified hearing problem. Burns (1968) suggested the average hearing level at 0·5, 1, 2 and 3 kHz, with a "threshold" of impairment at 30 dB, in contrast to the "three average threshold" of 25 dB. Other

---

* Now at Department of Social and Occupational Medicine, Welsh National School of Medicine, Cardiff.

combinations of frequencies have been discussed, among them the average at 0·5, 1, 2, 3, 4, 6 kHz (British Occupational Hygiene Society, 1970).

The female jute weavers with a constant noise exposure throughout their working lives, appeared to be a suitable, homogeneous population to ascertain whether the pure-tone audiogram, by any combination of frequencies, could give a valid measure of social impairment. In addition, any method of measurement derived from the weaving population, could be assessed using the control group, and those persons rejected from the main study because of otological abnormalities.

METHODS

Only a brief summary of the methods used in the collection of the data is presented. Full details are given in the paper comparing the matched groups of weavers and controls (Kell *et al.*, 1971).

Population

Records were available for 300 subjects. For the purposes of the study they were divided into 6 groups:

Group 1 Weavers with more than 20 years exposure (96 subjects with mean exposure 41·6 years to 100 dB(A)).

Group 2 Age- and residence-matched controls for Group 1 (96 subjects).

Group 3 Weavers with less than 20 years exposure (12 subjects).

Group 4 Age- and residence-matched controls for Group 3 (12 subjects).

Group 5 Extra controls not required in groups 2 and 4 (11 subjects).

Group 6 "Rejects"—a mixed group of weavers and controls with otological abnormalities or extraneous noise exposure (73 subjects).

Lists of retired and long-service employees were maintained in certain factories in Dundee. These lists provided the population of weavers in Dundee. In the other towns the weavers were obtained from the lists of the general practitioners. The controls were randomly selected from the lists of general practitioners in all areas, except for a small group of cleaners employed by the University of Dundee.

Pure-tone Audiometry

Pure-tone air conduction audiometry was performed in a sound-insulated room at frequencies 0·125, 0·25, 0·5, 1, 2, 3, 4, 6 and 8 kHz. In this part of the investigation the results for 0·125 kHz were not used. All measurements were made relative to British Standard 2497 (British Standards, 1954), with zero dB given by the following values for TDH39 earphones on a N.B.S. 9A artificial ear.

Frequency kHz	0·125	0·25	0·5	1	2	3	4	6	8
S.P.L. (dB)	50·5	30·5	15	10	9	10	10	23	15·5

Speech Audiometry
Speech audiometry was conducted using phonetically-balanced, mono-syllabic word lists (Fry, 1961). in the conventional manner using head-phones, and also in a semi-reverberant room against a noise background of 60 dB(A). The latter method was developed in conjunction with the University of Southampton (Acton, 1970). The measurements used were the sound levels at which 50 per cent of phonemes and 50 per cent of words were understood.

Questionnaire
In addition to the basic demographic data, the questionnaire covered the following areas.

1. Occupational history (with special reference to noise).
2. Difficulties in communication.
3. Difficulties in use of telephone.
4. Difficulties in use of radio and television.
5. Difficulties at public meetings.
6. Use of hearing aid.

Analysis
In deriving the measure of social impairment, the data from the group of weavers with more than 20 years' exposure were used. The matched control group was used to define the expected range in non-noise-exposed groups, in order to grade the various aspects of hearing con-sidered in the analysis.

The question for which an answer was sought may be stated, "Which combination of frequencies from the pure-tone audiogram would best distinguish 'deaf' and 'not deaf'?" Discriminant analysis (Rao, 1952; Anderson, 1958) may provide an answer, if known groups of "deaf" and "not deaf" are available. This is essentially a forward-looking technique, which defines a function from two known groups, to be applied to future individuals, in order to assign them to one of the two defining groups. Unfortunately, there is no absolute measure of social handicap which can be used in defining the groups. A suitable measure must be obtained from the social questionnaire.

Thus, the first stage of the analysis was to identify those factors on the questionnaire which provided the most sensitive measure of difficulty. For each factor the mean levels of the speech audiogram at the different degrees of difficulty were compared, using analysis of variance.

Those factors showing the most significant effects were then combined to give a single "social grade", using a system of weighting. "No difficulty" was scored 0, "maximum difficulty" scored 3, and any intermediate stages were scored 1 or 2. The distribution of the total scores in the weavers with more than 20 years' exposure was then compared with the matched control group, and five grades were established by grouping the scores such that the majority of the controls were in grades 0 and 1, and few, if any, were in grades 3 and 4.

Weavers in grades 0 and 1 were then defined as "not deaf". The "deaf" group consisted of the weavers in grades 3 and 4. The remainder grade 2, were not used in this part of the analysis, in an attempt to ensure a clear distinction between "deaf" and "not deaf". The puretone audiograms were then submitted to discriminant analysis using a computer program developed by the Biometric Laboratory of the University of Miami. The program was modified to work with the mean threshold of each subject, rather than the entire audiogram with the thresholds of right and left ears dealt with separately. This was done to produce a consistent pattern of frequencies in the final assessment. When the thresholds for individual ears were used the overall pattern was confused by an unpredictable selection of right and left at each frequency. The analysis gave coefficients to be applied to the threshold at each frequency, before adding to obtain the final discriminant score. Since this score was measured on an arbitrary scale the coefficients were adjusted to convert the score into the scale of an average hearing loss. Finally the coefficients were rounded off for ease of calculation.

In all of the work with questionnaire replies it was considered that the very subjective aspect of when a person reports "difficulty" made the "social grading" suspect. In an effort to overcome this, the terms "deaf" and "not deaf" were re-defined using the more objective results of speech audiometry. Weavers with results in the range achieved by the majority of the controls were considered "not deaf". Those with results considerably in excess of the controls were labelled "deaf". Again an intermediate group of weavers was discarded. The discriminant analysis was repeated to give a second discriminant function. The coefficients of the two functions were compared, and then averaged to give the final hearing loss index.

The properties of this index were investigated in all of the six groups in the study, and a description prepared of the difficulties experienced at the different levels of the index.

RESULTS AND DISCUSSION

Social Factors on Questionnaire

For the group of 96 weavers with more than 20 years' exposure, the replies to 10 different aspects of the hearing questionnaire were compared with the two main measurements from the speech audiogram, namely, dB level for 50 per cent phoneme score and for 50 per cent word score, both against a noise background. The mean levels of the speech audiogram measurements for each of the degrees of difficulty in the social factors were examined using analysis of variance and the F-test, as summarized in Table I.

The greatest separation of mean speech level was achieved by considering (a) face-to-face conversation with family and friends, (b) face-to-face conversation with strangers, (c) understanding of telephone conversation, and (d) own assessment of hearing. To a lesser extent, public meetings also showed significant differences in mean speech level. These were the factors which showed the largest differences when the weavers and controls were compared (Kell et al., 1971).

In almost all cases there was a stronger association between the 50 per cent word score and the social factors, than was found for the 50 per cent phoneme score. Indeed, for the 50 per cent word score, reactions of other people, preference for high volume on radio/T.V. and tendency to require radio/television volume higher than other members of household, also showed significant separation of speech levels.

Impairment Score Based on Social Factors

In deriving the score, four of the five factors showing the greatest association with the speech audiogram were used. The person's own assessment of hearing was considered to be too subjective for inclusion in the score. The weights assigned to the degrees of difficulty with the four main factors are shown in Table II. The total score from the social factors is in the range 0 (subject reporting no difficulty in all four factors) to 12 (subject reporting maximum difficulty in all four factors). The distribution of scores in the main weaver and control groups is shown in Table III. Five grades, labelled 0 to 4, were created. Of the 96 controls, 90 (94 per cent) had total scores less than 2 and this was taken as the upper limit of grade 1. Only one control scored more than 6, which was taken as the upper limit of grade 2. The number of subjects assigned to the five grades are also shown in Table III. Persons in grade 0 reported no difficulty on any of the factors. Minimum difficulty on not more than two factors was reported by those in grade 1. These minimal difficulties tended to be on communication against a background of noise. In grade 2, difficulty was experienced at minimum level on at

TABLE I

Comparison of Social Variables with Speech Audiogram

Mean sound pressure level (dB) for 50 per cent phoneme score and 50 per cent word score, both against a noise background, at different levels of difficulty reported in the social factors, for 96 weavers with more than 20 years' exposure to noise

Social variable	dB level for 50 per cent phonemes Difficulty			F and significance[1]	dB level for 50 per cent words Difficulty			F and significance[1]
	0	+	++		0	+	++	
Reactions of other people	68·8	70·5	72·5	2·1	73·1	75·3	79·0	6·2***
Communication with family and friends	68·1	71·8	77·9	16·3***	71·7	78·3	82·3	19·8***
Communication with strangers ..	67·6	71·4	75·7	11·9***	70·7	77·3	81·3	23·5***
Annoyed by shouting	71·6	75·3	75·0	2·5	76·7	79·0	80·1	2·1
Understanding of speech on telephone	68·1	69·6	75·6	16·2***	73·3	72·8	80·9	20·0***
Radio/T.V.—Preference for high volume	70·5	71·7	73·9	2·1	74·1	77·7	79·4	4·9**
Radio/T.V.—Preference for volume higher than others	69·0		72·1	2·8	73·5		78·6	8·7**
Radio/T.V.—Volume turned down by others	70·6	71·0	71·0	<1	76·0	75·0	77·3	<1
Public meetings	69·6	73·7	77·0	3·7*	74·2	78·6	85·5	5·6**
Own assessment of hearing	66·0	72·9	76·9	18·9***	71·3	77·9	82·6	19·3***

[1]Levels of significance: * P<0·05. **P<0·01. ***P<0·005.
Level of difficulty: O = none. + = moderate. + + = severe.

TABLE II

Scoring System for Impairment Based on Social Factors,
Individual Scores to be Added to Give Total Score

Factor	Degree of Difficulty	Score
Communication with family and friends	None	0
	Noise/Voices only	1
	At all times	3
Communication with strangers	None	0
	Noise/Voices only	1
	At all times	3
Telephone	None	0
	Sometimes	1
	At all times	3
Public Meetings	None	0
	but still sits at back	1
	moving to front	2
	stopped going	3

TABLE III

Distribution of Total Impairment Score, Defined from Social Factors,
in 96 Weavers and 96 Matched Controls, Showing Grouping
into Five Grades of Difficulty

Score	Grade	WEAVERS No. with each score	No. in each grade	CONTROLS No. in each score	No. in each grade
0	0	13	13	75	75
1	1	1	8	3	15
2		7		12	
3		6		3	
4		7		1	
5	2	9	28		5
6		6		1	
7		7		1	
8		12			
9	3	2	35		1
10		14			
11		10			
12	4	2	12		
TOTAL		96	96	96	96

least three factors. Anyone with maximum difficulty on a single factor was also in grade 2. In this grade almost all subjects experienced some difficulty in face-to-face conversation. Grade 3 contained those with maximum difficulty on at least two factors. Everyone in this grade was having difficulty in face-to-face conversation. Almost all were having some difficulty on all four factors. In grade 4 there was maximum difficulty on all factors, except possibly for public meetings where maximum was scored only when the subject no longer attended because of hearing difficulties. Many continued to attend such meetings, but admitted that they could no longer hear the speaker.

A second social grading was attempted, incorporating the other three factors showing an association with the speech audiogram. This did not improve the grading when the scores were compared with the speech audiogram, and was discarded.

Discriminant Function Based on Social Grading

In the discriminant analysis, 21 weavers (grades 0, 1) were in the "not deaf" group, and 47 (grades 3, 4) in the "deaf" group (Table III). The coefficients to be applied to the threshold at each audiometric frequency before adding to obtain the discriminant score were:

Frequency (Hz)	250	500	1 k	2 k	3 k	4 k	6 k	8 k
Coefficient	0	+1/6	−1/6	+7/6	+2/6	−6/6	+3/6	0

The function discriminates between "deaf" and "not deaf" at 40 dB.

Three of the 47 weavers in grades 3 and 4 gave values less than 40, and are thus "misclassified" by the function. Of the 21 weavers in grades 0 and 1, five gave values above 40, and are also "misclassified". This evaluation of the discriminant function assumes no "misclassification" by the subjects themselves due to under-reporting of difficulty by those in grades 0 and 1, or over-reporting by grades 3 and 4.

Discriminant Function Based on Speech Audiogram Grading

Most of the controls (92 per cent) reached the 50 per cent level in word score below 75 dB, and few (6 per cent) required levels in excess of 80 dB (Table IV). A second grading system, labelled O to IV, was defined in a similar way to that based on social scores, with the majority of the controls in grades O and I, and few in grades III and IV (Table IV). In the discriminant analysis, "deaf" was defined as levels of 50 per cent word scores of 80 dB or more (grade, III, IV) and "not deaf" as levels less than 75 dB (grades O, I). Using this definition there were 32

TABLE IV

Distribution of Sound Pressure Level (dB) for 50 Per Cent Word Score on Speech Audiogram in 96 Weavers and 96 Matched Controls, Showing Grouping into Five Grades of Difficulty

dB level	Grade	WEAVERS No. at dB level	WEAVERS No. in each grade	CONTROLS No. at dB level	CONTROLS No. in each grade
60–64	O	2	9	1	59
65–69		7		58	
70–74	I	19	19	17	17
75–79	II	20	20	2	2
80–84	III	22	22	3	3
85–89	IV	7	10	1	2
90+		3		1	
N.K.*		16	16	13	13
TOTAL		96	96	96	96

* Level not known—subject did not complete speech audiometry, or could not reach 50 per cent word score.

"deaf" and 28 "not deaf" weavers. The coefficients of the resulting function were:

Frequency (Hz)	250	500	1 k	2 k	3 k	4 k	6 k	8 k
Coefficient		0	0	+4/11	+8/11	−2/11	−3/11	+4/11	0

This function discriminates between "deaf" and "not deaf" at 37 dB. In this case, 3 of the "not deaf" and 2 of the "deaf" weavers were misclassified.

Derivation of Function for Hearing Loss Index

When the two discriminant functions were compared, some similarities were seen. Although the importance of the individual frequencies in the final assessment cannot be judged by examining the magnitude of the coefficients, the analysis did provide information on this point. In both cases the frequency 2 kHz was the most important, contributing two and a half times more than the next most important frequency to the discrimination. In the function based on the social grading this frequency was followed by 4 kHz and 6 kHz, while in the function based on the speech audiogram, 1 kHz, 6 kHz and 4 kHz were the next most important frequencies. When the coefficients were examined it was seen that only 2 kHz, 4 kHz and 6 kHz gave consistently positive or negative values. These similarities in the important frequencies suggested that the differences in the minor coefficients might be random deviations. Thus, the coefficients were averaged in an effort to produce a more stable result. Again the coefficients were rounded off to integers and a divisor introduced in order to retain a measurement in the scale of an average hearing loss. The resulting coefficients were:

Frequency (Hz)	250	500	1 k	2 k	3 k	4 k	6 k	8 k
Coefficient	0	0	0	$+1$	0	$-\frac{1}{2}$	$+\frac{1}{2}$	0

In this case the point for discrimination of "deaf" and "not deaf" is 45 dB.

This procedure has produced a function, the Dundee Index of hearing impairment, which is very suitable for practical work, since it is simple to apply to an audiogram. However, it must be shown to give satisfactory results in differentiating between those subjects who have difficulty with hearing and those who do not.

Properties of the Dundee Index of Hearing Impairment

The first item considered was the number of misclassifications of subjects in the original "deaf" and "not deaf" groups, defined both by social factors and by speech audiometry. The performance of the index in the control group was also examined in this context. Table V shows

TABLE V
Number of Misclassifications

Function	Known Social Grading				Known Speech Audiogram Grading			
	Weavers		Controls		Weavers		Controls	
	0, 1	3, 4	0, 1	3, 4	O,I	III,IV	O,I	III,IV
From social grading	5	3	5	0	6	0	1	1
From speech audiogram	5	6	3	0	3	2	0	1
Dundee Index	5	3	3	0	3	0	0	1

the numbers of subjects misclassified, i.e. assigned to the wrong group, by the index and two discriminant functions from which it was derived. In all cases the index equalled the performance of the better of the two original discriminant scores.

When examined in the same way, similar numbers of misclassifications by the index are found in the heterogeneous group of rejects (Table VI). Although the number of misclassifications based on the social grades was slightly higher, six of the ten misclassifications in grades 0 and 1 had scores just above the threshold of 45 dB.

Thus all groups were combined to give overall misclassification rates, for the index. Out of the 148 subjects with word score grades O or I, 8 (5·4 per cent) were misclassified, and of the 49 in grades III or IV,

TABLE VI
Number of Misclassifications by Dundee Index
(when compared with known social grading and speech audiogram grading in reject group)

	Number misclassified
Known social grade 0, 1	10
Known social grade 3, 4	2
Known speech audiogram grade O, I ..	4
Known speech audiogram grade III, IV ..	1

2 (4·1 per cent) were misclassified. When compared with the social grading, 20 (12·1 per cent) of the 165 subjects in grades 0 or 1, and 6 (8·0 per cent) of the 75 subjects in grades 3 or 4 were misclassified. It was expected that comparison with the social grading would lead to a higher rate of misclassification, particularly in grades 0 and 1, due to a reluctance to admit to difficulty, and to the wide subjective variation in the point at which "difficulty" is reported.

The distribution of the index in the three major groups in the study is shown in Fig. 1. Superimposed on the histograms is a shading to repre-

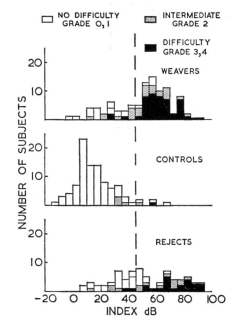

FIG. 1. Distribution of impairment index compared with grading based on questionnaire for the three main groups in the study. Index differentiates between "deaf" (grades 3 and 4) and "not deaf" (grades 0 and 1) at 45 dB.

sent the grading on the social scale derived from the questionnaire. Those subjects having difficulty (grades 3 and 4) were shaded black and mainly had indices more than 45 dB. Good hearing (grades 0 and 1), the unshaded areas, mainly occurred with indices less than 45 dB. The intermediate group (grade 2) which was not used in the derivation of the index, showed a wider variation but there was a tendency to have values greater than the threshold of 45 dB. The relation between index and social grade followed the same pattern in the three groups.

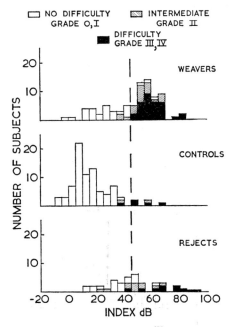

FIG. 2. Distribution of impairment index compared with grading based on speech audiogram for the three main groups in the study. Index differentiates between "deaf" (grades III and IV) and "not deaf" (grades O and I) at 45 dB.

A similarly consistent picture was obtained when the relationship between index and grading based on the speech audiogram was examined (see Fig. 2). In this case, a stronger association was seen, with little shading of any kind below 45 dB. Also a distinct threshold appeared. Examination of this diagram, particularly when the grades O and I were separated (Table VII) suggested the following grouping of the index as a measure of impairment:

(a) less than 25 dB   normal hearing
(b) 25–35   upper range of normality
(c) 35–45   beginning of impairment

(d) 45–55   definite impairment
(e) 55 +   severe impairment

Since the relation held in the control and reject groups in addition to the defining group of weavers, the index would appear to be generally applicable to hearing loss, and not simply a specific measure of noise-induced hearing loss.

Description of Grades of Impairment

The difficulty reported by subjects in the main areas considered is shown in Table VII for the different levels of the index. Since no difference in the performance of the index was noted in the different groups, all data has been combined in this table.

Normal Hearing—Index Less than 25 dB
Very few subjects reported difficulty, except for a small group having difficulty in conversation against a noise background. This can probably be explained by a varying interpretation of "difficulty". With a sufficiently loud background everyone has difficulty. No subjects required high levels on the speech audiogram.

Upper Range of Normality—Index in Range 25–35 dB
At this level the subjects began to notice some problems, particularly in conversation against a noise background and at public meetings. There was little evidence of difficulty in the speech audiogram, but there was a slight shift upwards in the level needed to achieve a 50 per cent word score, a shift still within the normal range.

Beginning of Impairment—Index in Range 35–45 dB
At this level more than half of the population were reporting difficulty in conversation against a noise background. One-third of the group were forced to move to the front at meetings. A very distinct shift to higher levels, outwith the normal range was seen in the speech audiogram. Also, at this level, other people began to notice and to comment on the deafness.

Definite Impairment—Index in Range 45–55 dB
At this level there was an increase in the number experiencing difficulty in conversation at all times, especially with strangers. There was an abrupt increase in the percentage having difficulty with the telephone, approximately half now reporting problems. The speech audiogram also showed definite changes, 38 per cent now being grade III or above, and only 16 per cent in grades O and I.

TABLE VII

Percentage of Subjects, in Each Grade of Impairment Defined by the Dundee Index

(reporting varying degrees of difficulty in the main social factors, and at each level of the socially-defined and speech-audiogram-defined gradings)

Area of difficulty	Difficulty	Index					
		<25	25–35	35–45	45–55	55–65	65 +
Face-to-face conversation with family and friends	At all times	0·9	5·6	8·3	8·6	44·4	48·1
	In noise only	11·1	38·9	58·3	65·7	33·3	48·1
Face-to-face conversation with strangers	At all times	1·7	8·3	12·5	28·6	61·1	65·4
	In noise only	11·1	36·1	54·2	48·6	22·2	32·7
Understanding of telephone	At all times	1·7	5·6	17·4	47·1	66·7	65·9
	"sometimes"	3·5	11·1	13·0	5·9	5·6	13·6
Public meetings	Stopped going	0·0	0·0	0·0	4·5	3·1	3·8
	Forced to move to front	3·7	7·7	33·3	22·7	34·4	34·6
	Not forced to move	1·9	23·1	25·0	40·9	46·9	50·0
Social Grading	4	0·0	0·0	0·0	5·7	16·7	17·3
	3	0·9	5·6	12·5	25·7	47·2	50·0
	2	3·4	27·8	50·0	34·3	22·2	26·9
	1	17·1	16·7	12·5	17·1	2·8	3·8
	0	78·6	50·0	25·0	17·1	11·1	1·9
Speech audiogram grading	4	0·0	0·0	0·0	12·9	19·4	30·0
	3	0·0	0·0	10·5	25·8	41·9	50·0
	2	1·0	3·7	31·6	45·2	29·0	20·0
	1	21·2	44·4	36·8	9·7	6·5	0·0
	0	77·9	51·9	21·1	6·5	3·2	0·0

Severe Impairment —Index More than 55 dB
More of the population reported difficulty at all times. Two-thirds had
difficulty with the telephone. More than 80 per cent had difficulty at
public meetings.

Comparison of the Dundee Index with Six Other Suggested Measures of Impairment

The measures used in this comparison were as follows:

Label	Definition Average of thresholds at
A	0·5, 1, 2 kHz
B	0·5, 1, 2, 3 kHz
C	0·5, 1, 2, 3, 4 kHz
D	1, 2, 3 kHz
E	0·5, 1, 2, 4 kHz
F	0·5, 1, 2, 3, 4, 6 kHz

The first factor examined was the number of misclassifications made
by each method in the "deaf" and "not deaf" groups, defined both by
social questionnaire and by speech audiometry. In this analysis the
results of all 300 subjects were used. Since the six averages do not
have thresholds for distinguishing between "deaf" and "not deaf" as
defined in this investigation, the distribution of each was examined and a
threshold defined which minimized the total number of misclassifications. Thus the index was compared with the best performance of each
of the other methods on this data.

In Table VIII is shown the minimum number of misclassifications
when compared with speech audiogram grading for each of the averages, together with the threshold at which this occurred. Also included
in the table is the number of misclassifications using the Dundee index.
The index gave the smallest number of misclassifications, and the
rates of misclassification were equal for "false positives" (assigning to
category "deaf" when "not deaf") and "false negatives" (assigning to
"not deaf" when "deaf"). Average F gave only slightly poorer results,
misclassifying one more person. Averages C and D gave the next lowest
total misclassifications, but C tended to give an excess of false positives
and D an excess of false negatives.

When the comparison was repeated for the socially defined "deaf"
and "not deaf" groups, the same threshold was retained for discrimination between "deaf" and "not deaf" (Table IX). This did not correspond to the minimum possible for two of the averages, A and D, whose

TABLE VIII

Misclassifications Using the Index Compared With Minimum Misclassifications for Six Average Hearing Losses

(based on 50 per cent word score on speech audiogram)

Average	Thresh-hold	Total misclassifications		Misclassifications in grades O, I		III, IV	
		No.	per cent	No.	per cent	No.	per cent
A	35	19	9·6	7	4·7	12	24·4
B	35	17	8·6	15	10·1	2	4·1
	40			9	6·1	8	16·3
C	40	14	7·1	12	8·1	2	4·1
D	45	13	6·6	6	4·1	7	14·3
E	35	15	7·6	14	9·5	1	2·0
F	45	11	5·6	9	6·1	2	4·1
DUNDEE INDEX	45	10	5·1	8	5·4	2	4·1

TABLE IX

Misclassifications Using the Index Compared With Misclassifications for Six Average Hearing Losses

(based on social grading from questionnaire, using same threshold as Table VIII)

Average	Thresh-hold	Total misclassifications		Misclassifications in grades 0, 1		3, 4	
		No.	per cent	No.	per cent	No.	per cent
A	35	37	15·4	20	12·1	17	22·7
	(30)	(36)	(15·0)	(29)	(17·6)	(7)	(9·3)
B	35	29	12·1	25	15·2	4	5·3
	40	31	12·9	19	11·5	12	16·0
C	40	26	10·8	22	13·3	4	5·3
D	45	28	11·7	17	10·3	11	14·7
	(40)	(26)	(10·8)	(20)	(12·1)	(6)	(8·0)
E	35	28	11·7	24	14·5	4	5·3
F	45	23	9·6	18	10·9	5	6·7
DUNDEE INDEX	45	26	10·8	20	12·1	6	8·0
	(50)	(18)	(7·5)	(11)	(6·7)	(7)	(9·3)

Figures in parentheses show true minimum misclassification.

true minima are also shown. All seven methods of assessment did less well in this comparison, average F giving the best result. The Dundee index and the averages C and D gave the next lowest total misclassifica tion. However, the index is being compared with the best possible performance of the other methods. If the true minimum of the index for differentiating socially defined "deaf" and "not deaf" is used, the Dundee index again gives the lowest number of misclassifications, 18 (7·5 per cent).

Thus, the index gave the best discrimination between "deaf" and "not deaf" in terms of misclassifications. Since the index was defined using these terms this might have been expected. However, the definition was made using only a subset of the records on which the evaluation has been made. The introduction of the control and reject data did not reduce the performance of the index.

The methods of assessing impairment were further compared by examining the mean level of each, in the five grades of hearing estab lished for the 50 per cent word score from the audiogram (Table X).

TABLE X

Mean Levels of Measures of Impairment in the Grades of Hearing Difficulty Defined by the Level for 50 Per Cent Word Score on the Speech Audiogram

| Average | O | GRADE OF DIFFICULTY | | | |
		I	II	III	IV
A	12·68	19·04	36·09	41·11	47·37
B	13·34	23·74	42·11	46·76	51·67
C	14·72	27·82	46·08	50·62	54·64
D	13·54	26·38	47·59	53·36	56·79
E	14·65	25·22	42·69	47·34	52·16
F	16·63	30·44	49·12	53·66	56·99
INDEX	16·12	25·73	51·25	60·62	62·26

Average F and the Dundee index showed the greatest differences between the grades. The mean levels of these two best measures are shown in Fig. 3, as differences from the mean level in the first grade. The index had the lowest mean for the "not deaf" (50 per cent word score levels in the range 70–75 dB) and the highest mean in the "deaf" (50 per cent word score level more than 80 dB). The index showed the largest differences between the extreme groups, and thus the best discrimination of hearing difficulties.

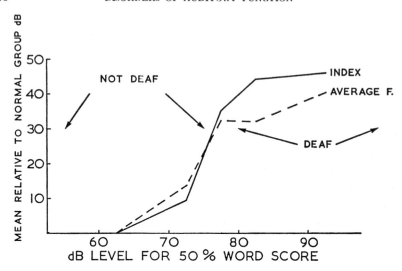

FIG. 3. Mean level of the two "best" measures of impairment compared with dB level for 50 per cent word score in the speech audiogram. Means are shown as differences from the mean level in the group with normal speech audiogram results. "Index" is (threshold at 2 kHz) $- \frac{1}{2}$ (threshold at 4 kHz) $+ \frac{1}{2}$ (threshold at 6 kHz), and "average F" is average of thresholds at 0·5, 1, 2, 3, 4 and 6 kHz.

THE ROLE OF THE THRESHOLDS AT 4kHz AND 6kHz IN THE INDEX

Since the threshold at 2 kHz was the important part of the index, an examination of the effect of the other two thresholds was made. The index was divided into two components:

$$(a) \ 2 \text{ kHz}, \qquad (b) \ \tfrac{1}{2}(6 \text{ kHz–4 kHz})$$

These components were calculated for each subject. Examination of the effects of the components revealed that the component $\frac{1}{2}(6$ kHz–4 kHz) takes account of the shape of the audiogram and distinguishes between those audiograms where there is a steadily increasing loss with increasing frequency (component positive), and those where the maximum loss is at 4 kHz with an improvement in threshold at the higher frequencies (component negative). Some examples illustrating the effect of the component $\frac{1}{2}(6$ kHz–4 kHz) are shown in Figs. 4, 5 and 6.

Subjects 38 and 46 (Fig. 4). These subjects are of the same age and have similar thresholds at 2 kHz, but subject 46 has considerably poorer hearing when tested using speech audiometry. The threshold at 2 kHz alone cannot distinguish between these subjects, nor can the averages discussed above which assess subject 38 as having the poorer hearing.

The inclusion of the component utilizing the thresholds at 4 kHz and 6 kHz enables the index to identify correctly the subject with poorer hearing.

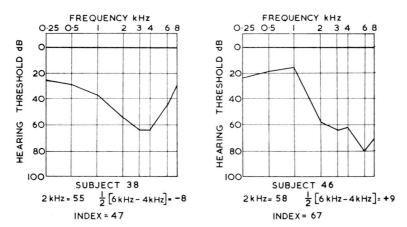

FIG. 4. Effect of the component $\frac{1}{2}$(6 kHz–4 kHz) on the index for subjects of the same age with similar thresholds at 2 kHz, where subject 46 has poorer hearing than subject 38 when assessed using speech audiometry.

Subjects 28 and 314 (Fig. 5). Here the thresholds at 2 kHz are different but the subjects give the same response to speech audiometry. By taking account of the shapes of the audiograms the index assesses these subjects as having the same degree of deafness.

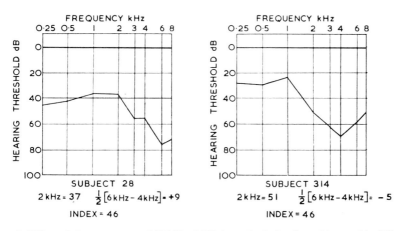

FIG. 5. Effect of the component $\frac{1}{2}$(6 kHz–4 kHz) on the index for subjects with different thresholds at 2 kHz but similar hearing when assessed using speech audiometry.

L

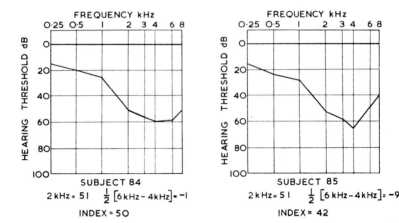

FIG. 6. Effect of the component $\frac{1}{2}$(6 kHz–4 kHz) on the index for subjects with similar thresholds at 2 kHz, but subject 84 has the poorer hearing when assessed using speech audiometry.

Subjects 84 and 85 (Fig. 6). In this case the difference between the audiograms is less extreme. The threshold at 2 kHz and the other measures of deafness discussed above give the same score to these subjects, but subject 84 gives very much poorer results on the speech audiogram. The larger correction for shape for subject 85 successfully identifies the subject with better hearing.

CONCLUSIONS

1. An index for the assessment of hearing impairment from the pure tone air conduction audiogram was derived by examining groups of "deaf" and "not deaf" weavers, the groups being defined both in terms of social variables and speech audiometry. The composition of the Dundee index was: (threshold at 2 kHz) − $\frac{1}{2}$ (threshold at 4 kHz) + $\frac{1}{2}$ (threshold at 6 kHz).

In each case the threshold is the average of the two ears.

2. The limits of the Dundee index for different levels of impairment were:

less than 25 dB	normal hearing
25–35	upper range of normality
35–45	beginning of impairment
45–55	definite impairment
55 +	severe impairment

3. The Dundee index successfully assessed hearing impairment in groups of controls and persons with hearing abnormalities in addition to the population of weavers on which the derivation was carried out.

4. The Dundee index was compared with six other suggested measures of impairment based on averages of various frequencies of the audiogram. The index made fewer misclassifications than the others, and showed a greater difference in mean level between the extreme groups.

SUMMARY

An index for the assessment of hearing impairment from the pure-tone air conduction audiogram was derived by examining groups of "deaf" and "not deaf" weavers, the groups being defined both in terms of social variables and of the speech audiogram. The composition of the Dundee index was:

$$(\text{threshold at } 2 \text{ kHz}) - \tfrac{1}{2} (\text{threshold at } 4 \text{ kHz}) + \tfrac{1}{2} (\text{threshold at } 6 \text{ kHz})$$

Limits for levels of impairment were defined. The index was tested on two other populations and was successful in assessing impairment. When compared with other suggested measures of impairment the index made fewer misclassifications and showed a greater difference in mean level between the extreme groups.

ACKNOWLEDGEMENTS

This study was carried out under grants from the Advisory Committee for Medical Research (R.L.K.) and the Medical Research Council (W.T. and W.I.A.).

Our thanks are due to Miss C. French for the computer programming. Finally we would like to thank the members of the general population of Dundee and district who co-operated in this study, and the weavers, without whom the investigation could not have been carried out.

REFERENCES

Acton, W. I. (1970). Speech intelligibility in a background noise and noise-induced hearing loss. *Ergonomics*, **13**, 546–554.

Anderson, T. W. (1958). "An Introduction to Multivariate Statistical Analysis". pp. 126–138, Wiley, New York.

British Occupational Hygiene Society Committee on Hygiene Standards (1971). Hygiene standard for Wide Band Noise, *Ann. Occ. Hyg.*, **14**, 2, 57–64.

Burns, W. (1968). "Noise and Man". J. Murray, London.

Davis, H., Kranz, F. W. (1964). The international standard reference zero for pure-tone audiometers and its relation to the evaluation of impairment of hearing. *J. Speech Hearing Res.*, **7**, 7–16.

Fox, M. S. (1965). Comparative provisions for occupational hearing loss. *Arch. Otolaryng.*, **81**, 257–260.

Fry, D. B. (1961). Word and sentence tests in use in speech audiometry. *Lancet*, **2**, 197–199.

Glorig, A. (1959). Hearing conservation, past and future. *Trans. Am. Acad. Ophthal. Otolaryng.*, **63**. Suppl. 24–33.

Glorig, A. (1966). Audiometric reference levels. *Laryngoscope*, **76**, 842–849.

High, W. S., Fairbanks, G. and Glorig, A. (1964). Scale for self-assessment of hearing handicap. *J. Speech Hearing Dis.*, **29**, 215–230.

Hinchcliffe, R. (1959). The threshold of hearing as a function of age. *Acustica*, **9**, 303–308.

Kell, R. L., Pearson, J. C. G. and Taylor, W. (1970). Hearing thresholds of an island population in North Scotland. *Int. Audiol.*, **9**, 334–349.

Kell, R. L., Pearson, J. C. G., Acton, W. I. and Taylor, W. (1971). Social effects of hearing loss due to weaving noise. *In* "Occupational Hearing Loss" (D. W. Robinson, ed.), Academic Press, London and New York.

Rao, C. R. (1952). "Advanced Statistical Methods in Biometric Research". pp. 237–238; 246–248. Wiley, New York,

Taylor, W., Pearson, J., Mair, A. and Burns, W. (1965). Study of noise and hearing in jute weaving. *J. acoust. Soc. Am.*, **38**, 113–120.

Taylor, W., Pearson, J. and Mair A. (1967). Hearing thresholds of a non-noise-exposed population in Dundee. *Br. J. Ind. Med.*, **24**, 114–122.

The normal threshold of hearing for pure tones by earphone listening. British Standards Institution, London. B.S. 2497 (1954).

Noise, the Abnormal Ear and the Jet Engine

D. L. CHADWICK

*Department of Otolaryngology, The University,
Manchester, England*

What happens to the healthy ear in noise is well known. How the diseased ear reacts is less clearly understood.

Jet engine development has added a new dimension to the noises assaulting the hearing of modern man. At the present time it is not uncommon to be confronted with patients exposed to noise of this nature. Under conditions of such undue acoustic insult, particularly when the ear has already been the subject of previous pathological attack, the results caused by intense jet-engine noise upon hearing may frequently be more devastating than in otherwise normal ears.

Any protective cover provided by pathological processes may be overriden by the intense stimulation of this type of noise. Even in normal ears marked hearing impairment can occur.

The audiograms for left and right ears of a middle-aged employee, showed a marked permanent threshold shift after two years jet-engine noise exposure.

This brief report is based on two studies. Firstly a survey of jet-engine workers; secondly, the investigation of patients with abnormal ears and evidence of noise-induced hearing loss, employed in the gas-turbine industry and in other noise-hazardous environments.

The practical implications relate to the desirability or otherwise of employing personnel with ears already impaired in noisy industrial processes; the steps to be taken when such individuals are already found working in oto-traumatic situations and the advice to be given to people with hearing defects which are remedial by surgery who are exposed to noise, both before and after operative intervention.

In studying the development of noise-induced hearing loss, consideration must be given to the noise, the individual, and the ear.

NOISE

With regard to noise, the parameters of frequency, intensity, duration and character, whether continuous, intermittent, impulsive, steady-state, etc., must be evaluated.

Jet noise is a very complex modality compounded of a continuous background noise of high intensity with variable rising and falling characteristics, punctuated by intermittent impulsive peaks of much greater sound pressure levels (Eldredge, 1960).

THE INDIVIDUAL

Where the human element is concerned, age, individual susceptibility, general health, and possibly sex, are relevant factors.

THE EAR

When considering the ear, pathological conditions introduce additional attributes which must be studied to determine the manner in which the ear's normal response to noise may be modified. Certain disease processes may afford increased protection to the cochlea when assaulted by noise.

In other instances, the adverse effects of high intensity sound stimulation may be exaggerated in the presence of otological abnormalities.

The purpose of this presentation is to consider those features which may alter the reaction of the inner ear to noise, those disorders likely to result in increased safety, and those which may cause exaggerated damage to the organ of Corti.

These remarks will be illustrated by reference to cases studied in clinical practice, including examination of some 300 patients with presumptive evidence of noise-induced hearing loss, of whom approximately 16 per cent had additional aural pathology.

Numerous factors within the ear may modify the harmful effects of noise. Briefly, these may be grouped together as faults in the normal sound-conducting transducer mechanism, including impaired resonance in the mastoid cells; and defects in the sensori-neural receptor elements.

External and Middle Ear

The transmission of sound waves across the middle ear may be interfered with as a result of meatal obstruction, tympanic perforations, altered drum mobility, middle ear granulations, cholesteatoma, fluid, adhesions and tympanosclerosis; the extent of mastoid pneumatization, the degree of stapes fixation, malfunction of the auditory tube and the activity of the intra-tympanic muscles.

Inner Ear

Influences to be considered within the inner ear include the tension of the endolymph, the integrity of the neurosensory epithelium and Corti's organ, and the state of the auditory nerve fibres and ganglia.

Aural Pathology

Certain forms of aural pathology may protect the cochlea from noise damage.

In general, it has been considered that conductive lesions provide additional protective cover for the cochlea, particularly where there is ankylosis of the stapedial footplate.

Bunch (1937) one of the pioneers of audiology, considered middle ear adhesions to exert a protective effect and Glorig's (1958) conception of the 'built-in ear-plug' provided by conductive deafness is well known.

Otitis Media

A protective effect attributed to obsolete otitis media was demonstrated in the audiogram of a jet engine worker. His hearing after two years' exposure showed in fact a slight improvement over the initial threshold. Over the same period, the opposite ear, with a normal drum, showed permanent deterioration in hearing, of sensori-neural type.

Adhesions involving the round and oval window regions have been considered a possible reason for protection of the inner ear in otitis media (Mounier-Kuhn, 1959). It has, however, been pointed out that although protection occurs in some cases, in others the effects of middle-ear suppuration constitute an aggravating factor (Hustin, 1961). There is more likelihood of cochlear damage when the mastoid process is sclerotic than when it is well pneumatized. This is considered due to loss of the normal dampening action of the mastoid cells on movements of the tympanic membrane (Onchi, 1966).

A case in point was a 57-year-old Aircraft Inspector. He complained of deafness and tinnitus, mainly in the right ear. The eardrums were intact and stapedius muscle reflexes normal. Radiologically the left mastoid process showed abundant pneumatization. On the right, pneumatization of the mastoid cells was much reduced and pure-tone audiograms demonstrated a marked "acoustic dip" in the right ear at 4 kHz.

Since mastoid sclerosis is a common accompaniment of chronic middle-ear disease, this is one possible explanation of the equivocal findings recorded in otitis media.

In some instances a built-in protective ear-plug appears to have been operative; in others, the traumatic effects of noise have been enhanced.

Severe bilateral perceptive deafness was observed in a man with inactive otitis media in both ears, after two years' jet-engine exposure. He was still capable of recording an appreciable temporary threshold shift at the end of a day's work.

A blacksmith presented with an aural polyp After removal, this was found to have arisen from a marginal perforation in the postero-superior quadrant of the drum. His audiogram showed reasonable bone conduction in this ear. In the opposite ear, which had a normal tympanic membrane, there was a severe high tone deafness, air and bone conduction being both markedly reduced. This suggests that in the infected ear, the aural polyp had cushioned the blows from his blacksmith's anvil and lessened the acoustic damage to the cochlea on this side.

Otosclerosis

Otosclerosis comes into a somewhat different category since the essential lesion results in fixation of the stapedial footplate in the oval window.

If an individual is exposed to noise before the stapes has become completely fixed, we may well find the presence of a classical "noise notch" around 4 kHz, in addition to the otosclerotic conductive loss in the lower frequencies. When ankylosis of the stapes occurs before employment in noise, the picture is frequently that of a pure conductive' deafness with no "acoustic dip"; suggesting that cochlear protection has been achieved.

Should surgical correction of otosclerotic deafness be advised in people exposed to noise?

When stapes mobilization was the operation of choice, a subsequent 3 kHz dip was reported not infrequently (Fletcher and King, 1963; Steffen et al., 1963; Lehnhardt, 1967).

What is the position today, when some form of stapedectomy is now the procedure practised almost universally?

In the early days of this technique, it was suggested that noise-damage to the cochlear might be induced by the use of a drill (Schuknecht and Tonndorf, 1960). Severe inner ear changes and substantial threshold shifts in stapedectomized patients working in noise were reported (Kos, 1962; Sagardia, 1963; Bull, 1966).

On the other hand, Gibb (1963) has reported cases showing no deterioration and other similar results have been recorded (Ferris, 1965, 1967). My own experience with stapedectomized cotton weavers is largely in line with these findings.

Nevertheless it seems prudent to concur with the view that post-stapedectomized ears should be adequately protected when exposed to sound pressure levels known to be hazardous to the cochlea (Taylor and Williams, 1966).

Consideration must be given to the possible protective role of the stapedius muscle reflex. The stapedius tendon is, of course, divided during stapedectomy.

With a mobile stapes it has been found that contraction of the stapedius muscle in response to noise will prevent excessive excursions of the footplate, thereby reducing the damaging effects of noise on the inner ear (Fletcher and Riopelle, 1963).

It has been suggested that this fact might be utilized in reducing the temporary threshold shifts caused by impulse noise. A non-hazardous noise, sufficient to produce contraction of the stapedius muscle applied a few μsec before exposure to impulse noise may thereby protec tthe cochlea (Coles, 1967; Fletcher and Loeb, 1962).

SOME ILLUSTRATIVE STAPEDECTOMIES

Reference will now be made to some cases of stapedectomy working in noise.

The audiograms of a middle-aged weaver, showed initial complete closure of the air-bone gap, followed subsequently by slight elevation of the air-conduction threshold following her return to work. There was also a sizeable pre-operative high-tone loss. She started work in the mill when she was 15 years of age.

Conversely, a young male otosclerotic first became aware of the handicap of deafness when exposed to the noise of a new printing press.

Stapedectomy resulted in closure of the air-bone gap at the lowest frequencies and also in a considerable high-tone loss. Ear protectors were supplied but he soon abandoned them, claiming that these prevented him from detecting fine changes in the noise of his machine whilst it was running. Following this, further deterioration in his hearing ensued.

Two further cases illustrate the diagnostic difficulties which may be encountered and the fact that sometimes more than one form of pathology may be present.

In one instance, obsolete otitis media and otosclerosis co-existed; in the other, otosclerosis was associated with sclerotic mastoids.

The first man, 45 years old, had never heard well, had a family history of otosclerosis and his whole working life had been spent in noise, including jet-engine noise. There was no known history of otitis media, but X-ray examination showed the right mastoid poorly pneumatized compared with the left.

Audiograms showed a mixed deafness, with air conduction worse right than left, but with better bone conduction in this ear. Both stapedius muscle reflexes were absent.

A right tympanotomy revealed otosclerotic fixation of the stapes. Necrosis of the long process of the incus which was surrounded by adhesions provided evidence of previous middle-ear inflammation.

Stapedectomy was performed and he returned to his current employment as a jet-engine fitter.

In a short time bone conduction in his operated ear, previously the better of the two, deteriorated to approximately the same level as that in the unoperated ear.

It is interesting to speculate whether his long-standing adhesions may have provided some protection to the cochlea during his previous noise exposure.

Another otosclerotic whose occupation involved the use of a pneumatic drill underwent a right stapedectomy. Radiologically both mastoids were sclerotic and poorly pneumatized. Pre-operatively both ears showed considerable high-tone loss. Seven years after his stapedectomy, during which time he had continued in the same employment, the unoperated ear showed a much more marked high-tone deterioration than did the stapedectomized ear.

Inner-ear Lesions

With regard to inner-ear lesions, the behaviour on exposure to noise is also variable. Contrary opinions have again been expressed.

Apart from endolymphatic hydrops, sensori-neural deafness, other than that associated with noise or presbycusis, has been considered by some authors to be less susceptible to aggravation by noise than normal (Glorig, 1958; Hinchcliffe, 1967).

The opposing view, that early and rapid development of occupational hearing loss may occur in this type of deafness, has also been expressed (Sagardia, 1968).

A girl, unaware of any hearing disability when she left school, soon noticed she was severely handicapped after working for a short time in a noisy machine shop.

Her audiogram showed a severe high-tone sensori-neural deafness and there was found to be a family history of congenital inner-ear deafness.

An engineer with a mild sensori-neural deafness showed an accelerated rate of increase in his deafness during a two-year period of exposure to gas-turbine noise.

Similarly, a young man, treated with streptomycin 10 years previously, was exposed to intense jet-engine test-bed noise for 18 months.

During this period a very marked permanent elevation in his hearing threshold occurred.

SUMMARY AND CONCLUSIONS

The impact of noise on an already impaired organ of hearing may produce a variety of responses.

A study of some of the problems involved, with particular reference to jet-engine noise, illustrated by a number of case reports has been presented. It is hoped that further research into this subject may be stimulated and additional data recorded in an attempt further to elucidate the behaviour of the pathological ear in noise.

REFERENCES

Bull, T. R. (1966). *J. Laryng.*, **80**, 631.
Bunch, C. C. (1937). *Laryngoscope*, **47**, 615.
Coles, R. R. A. (1967). *Ann. occup. Hyg.*, **10**, 387.
Eldredge, D. H. (1960). *Laryngoscope*, **70**, 373.
Ferris, K. (1965). *J. Laryng.*, **79**, 881.
Ferris, K. (1967). *J. Laryng.*, **81**, 613.
Fletcher, J. L. and King, W. P. (1963). *Ann. Otol. St. Louis*, **72**, 900.
Fletcher, J. L. and Loeb, M. (1962). *Acta Otolaryng.*, **54**, 33.
Fletcher, J. L. and Riopelle, A. J. (1960). *J. acoust. Soc. Am.*, **32**, 401.
Gibb, A. G. (1963). *J. Laryng.*, **78**, 561.
Glorig, A. (1958). "Noise and Your Ear". p. 102. Grune and Stratton, New York.
Hinchcliffe, R. (1967). *Proc. R. Soc. Med.*, **60**, 1111.
Hustin, A. (1961). *Acta O.R.L. Belg.*, **15**, 383.
Kos, C. M. (1962). "Otosclerosis". (ed. H. F. Schuknecht), p. 497, London.
Lehnhardt, E. (1967). *Int. Audiol.*, **6**, 86.
Mounier-Kuhn, P. (1959). "Colloque sur le Bruit", Paris.
Onchi, Y. (1966). *Proc. VIII Congr. int. Oto-rhino-laryng.*, 211.
Sagardia, J. R. M. (1963). *Int. Audiol.*, **2**, 247.
Sagardia, J. R. M. (1968). *Int. Audiol.*, **7**, 121.
Schuknecht, H. F. and Tonndorf, J. (1960). *Laryngoscope*, **70**, 479.
Steffen, T. N., Nixon, J. C. and Glorig, A. (1963). *Laryngoscope*, **73**, 1044.
Taylor, G. D. and Williams, E. (1966). *Laryngoscope*, **76**. 863.

The Extent and Severity of Occupational Deafness Among Men Employed as Drop Forgers

G. R. C. ATHERLEY

Safety and Hygiene Group, University of Aston in Birmingham, Birmingham, England

The purposes of this paper are to give an estimate of the numbers of men employed in drop forging who are likely to have symptoms of occupational deafness, and to indicate the numbers of men that are likely to be severely affected by it.

BACKGROUND

In drop forging a piece of hot metal is squeezed between two halves of a die that are brought together with a sharp blow often with the fall of a heavy weight as the driving force. Figure 1 shows the main features of a drop hammer: the lower half of the die is attached to a firm base and the upper half is secured by a wedge to the heavy weight known as the tup. This slides between two vertical pillars; a lifting mechanism raises it to the top of the pillars. An operator controls the fall of the tup so that each forging receives the correct number of blows at the right force.

Figure 2 shows drop forge men at work. The stamper's helper holds the billet of hot metal in tongs (seen lying on the drum in the foreground of the picture). The fall of the tup produces an extremely loud impact sound. The impacts grow progressively louder as the forging approaches its final shape; the men speak of the kissing of the dies.

The impacts are very interesting from the acoustical point of view. Impacts from the collision of solids generally have a distinctive waveform (Fig. 3). The envelope has an exponential outline; in the figure this is especially clear because the train of impacts has been synthesized electronically. Three quantities can be deduced from a picture of a waveform: the peak height, the decay time and the total number of impacts in a given period of time. It has been shown (Martin, 1970;

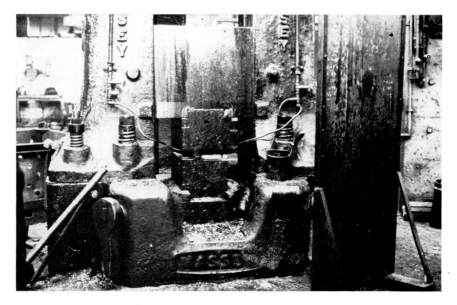

FIG. 1.

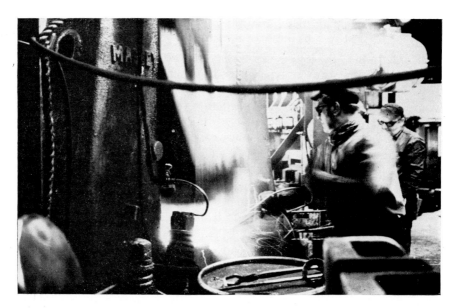

FIG. 2.

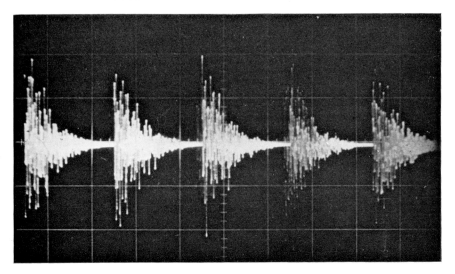

FIG. 3.

Atherley and Martin, 1971) that the three quantities can be used to calculate the sound energy in a train of pulses (further information about this is given as an appendix to this paper). From the calculations it is possible to obtain a measure of a quantity of considerable practical importance—the equivalent-continuous noise level (ECNL).

The British Occupational Hygiene Society's Hygiene Standard for Wide-band Noise (1971) describes ECNL.* This is the level of continuous noise in dB(A) which in the course of an eight-hour day would cause the same amount of sound energy to be received as that due to the actual noise over a typical day.

It is now widely accepted—on the basis of the work by Burns and Robinson (1970)—that ECNL can be used to predict the degree of danger from continuous noise. This is true over a wide range of sound levels and exposure durations.

We deduced (Atherley and Martin, 1971) the ECNLs associated with drop forges that we studied. We found that these ECNLs related mathematically to the hearing levels we actually measured on drop forgers. The mathematical expression is that given by Robinson (1968) and Robinson and Cook (1968).

The only noise for which the energy principle cannot yet be assumed is impulse noise caused by the sudden expansion of gases—gunfire is one example. In out-of-doors conditions this has a different waveform

* Since this was written the Department of Employment has published the Code of Practice for reducing the exposure of employed persons to noise; this defines equivalent-continuous sound level.

from that of impact noise. As knowledge stands at the time of writing the method of measurement described by Coles and Rice (1971) is the best approach for impulse noise.

THE PRESENT STUDY

It should be mentioned that all three of the quantities present difficulties in measurement under field conditions; this is a matter which has been discussed elsewhere (Hempstock *et al.*, 1972; Martin and Atherley, 1972). In particular it is not always easy to estimate how many impacts the men have been exposed to. Information from the work study and production departments is needed to make the calculations of ECNL. Measurements of noise are one problem: measurements of men's exposure are another.

I have used ECNL = 118 dB(A) for the present estimation. This is one of the highest figures to come out of the various surveys done by my colleagues and me. It represents a very noisy forge that is consistently operated at a high rate. Of course not all forges are associated with an ECNL as high as this so my estimates may err on the high side of the true figures.

The first step in my calculation was to find the noise immission level as described by Robinson. This quantity is given by the expression:

$$\text{NIL (in dB)} = \text{ECNL} + 10 \log_{10} Y/1$$

where Y is the years of exposure to the ECNL in question.

The years of exposure for the workforce of drop forgers has to be estimated because there is no direct information available. I have assumed that, as a group, drop forgers never change to other kinds of work. But in practice there must be some men who leave the industry to take up jobs that are quieter. Also there must be some who are recruited to drop forging after several years of work in quiet jobs. In the absence of information about these trends I have been obliged to assume that the effects of these changes will balance each other out. I have proceeded on the basis that men in the age decade 20–29 years have worked for an average of 10 years in drop forging, those in the 30–39 decade have done 20 years, and so on. The NILs can now be calculated (Table I).

TABLE I

Calculated NILs for Drop Forgers

Age range (yr)	20–29	30–39	40–49	50–59	60–64	65+
Calculated NILs (dB) for drop forgers	128	131	133	134	134·5	135

The next step was to find out how many drop forgers there are, and how many there are at various points in the age span.

The *Employment and Productivity Gazette* (1969) gives information about the size of workforce in various industries. From these figures I deduce that about 7,200 are employed actually operating drop forges. The Drop Forging Research Association (1971) estimates that no more than 8,000 men are employed in this way. Thus it seems likely that the *Gazette*'s figures are reasonably realistic.

The age structure was not as easy to determine. No direct information is available so an estimate had to be made. The *Gazette* (1970) gives the numbers of men that fall into seven decades and semi-decades that span 15–65 years of age. Information is available for 25 major categories of industry but it is not sufficiently detailed for the drop forgers to be separated. From the information that is given, the numbers in the decades can be expressed as a percentage of the total work force. When this is done it can be seen that there are no gross differences in age distribution from one industry to another. Thus it is reasonable to take the overall percentages in order to deduce the numbers of drop forgers in the decades. It should be noted that no account is taken of men in the semi-decade 15–19. This is because their exposure to drop forging noise will have been small. The various figures relating to drop forging are shown in Table I.

Next, the *Hygiene Standard* (1971) was consulted. This gives a graph showing the relation between NIL and percentages of a population having symptoms of occupational deafness at the end of a working life-time. Table II shows the percentages relating to the NILs shown in

TABLE II

Estimated Age Structure of Workforce of Drop Forgers Totalling 7,200 Men

Age range (yr)	20–29	30–39	40–49	50–59	60–64	65+
P (per cent)*	21	19	22	19	8	2·5
No. of men (to nearest 10)	1,510	1,370	1,580	1,370	580	180

*P is the percentage of the workforce in the age range; it is derived from figures for total male workforce in the U.K. (see text).

Table I. The percentages that are shown in the *Hygiene Standard* were calculated from the number of people whose score on a hearing questionnaire exceeded a criterion. The criterion was based upon the lowest scores of a group of people attending a hearing aid clinic (for further

M

information on hearing questionnaires see Atherley and Noble, 1971; Kell *et al.*, 1971).

It should be pointed out that the *Hygiene Standard*'s percentages relate to a working population at the end of its working lifetime. Relatively young people with high noise immission levels may not be affected as badly as the *Hygiene Standard*'s data appear to predict.

Table II shows the numbers of men in the various age groupings estimated to have symptoms of occupational deafness. These figures were, of course, derived by the method just described. It can be seen that out of a total workforce of 7,200 men something like 2,900 (40 per cent) are likely to have symptoms of occupational deafness. At first sight these appear to be alarmingly high figures but they should be interpreted with caution. We should remember that drop forging is one of the very noisiest of industries and, so far, no indication has been given of the likely severity of the symptoms.

TABLE III

Estimated Numbers of Men with Symptoms of Occupational Deafness

Age range (yr)	20–29	30–39	40–49	50–59	60–64	65+
NIL (dB)*	128	131	133	134	134·5	135
S (per cent)*	35	42	47	50	52	53
No. of men (to nearest 10)	530	570	740	680	300	100
	Grand total 2,900 (to nearest 100)					

*S is the percentage of a population who would show symptoms of occupational deafness (see text).

SEVERITY OF SYMPTOMS

The clinical picture of occupational deafness among drop forgers has been studied (Atherley and Noble, 1971); about half of those with symptoms—about 1,500 men—will have symptoms no more severe than this:

> In conversation with groups of people both at home and outside some difficulty is experienced from time to time. Conversation with one person outside may also present occasional difficulty but there is none at home. On occasion wrong answers are given and sometimes, not often, speech in TV plays appears indistinct. Certain domestic sounds such as the clock ticking may be missed. The man is aware that his hearing is less than normal but at the same time he is not prepared to say that his hearing is abnormal for his age.

About a quarter of those with symptoms—about 700 men—will have symptoms as severe as this:

Difficulty in conversation, individual and group, at home, work or outside is a common occurrence. There is difficulty in hearing what is said at public meetings. The man finds that people fail to speak clearly and very often speech on TV is indistinct. The sounds of home and street are often missed and difficulty is sometimes experienced in the perception of direction and distance of sound. He is aware that his hearing is not normal although he claims his difficulty imposes no restriction on his social or personal life. He knows that other people notice his difficulty in hearing. He quite often becomes irritated with himself because he is unable to follow conversations and there are occasions when he feels cut off. He does get tinnitus but it does not trouble him.

CONCLUSION

On the present evidence it seems that no more than about 10 per cent of the drop forgers are likely to be suffering from occupational deafness of severe degree.

REFERENCES

Atherley, G. R. C. and Martin, A. M. (1971). Equivalent-continuous Noise Level as a Measure of Injury from Impact and Impulse Noise, *Ann. Occupat. Hyg.*, **14**, 11–28.

Atherley, G. R. C. and Noble, W. G. (1971). Clinical picture of occupational hearing loss obtained with the hearing measurement scale. *In* "Occupational Hearing Loss" (ed. D. W. Robinson), Academic Press, London.

British Occupational Hygiene Society (1971). "Hygiene Standard for Wide-band Noise," Pergamon Press, Oxford.

Burns, W. and Robinson, D. W. (1970). "Hearing and Noise in Industry", H.M.S.O., London.

Coles, R. R. A. and Rice, C. G. (1971). Assessment of risk of hearing loss due to impulse noise. *In* "Occupational Hearing Loss" (ed. D. W. Robinson), Academic Press, London.

Employment and Productivity Gazette (1969). "Occupations of Employees in Manufacturing Industries", May 1968, LXXVII, 14–26.

Employment and Productivity Gazette (1970). "Numbers of Employees in Great Britain", June 1969, LXXVIII, 581.

Hempstock, T. I., Powell, J. A. and Else, D. (1972). (In press.)

Kell, R. L., Pearson, J. C. G., Acton, W. I. and Taylor, W. (1971). Social effects of hearing loss due to weaving noise. *In* "Occupational Hearing Loss" (ed. D. W. Robinson), Academic Press, London.

Martin, A. M. (1970), Industrial Impact Noise and Hearing, Ph.D. Thesis, University of Salford.

Martin, A. M. and Atherley, G. R. C. (1972). (In press.)

Robinson, D. W. (1968). "The Relationship Between Hearing Loss and Noise Exposure", NPL Aero Report AC32, National Physical Laboratory, England.

Robinson, D. W. and Cook, J. P. (1968). "The Quantification of Noise Exposure", NPL Aero Report AC32, National Physical Laboratory, England.

APPENDIX

Expression for the calculation of the equivalent-continuous noise level (ECNL) in dB(A) for a train of exponentially decaying impacts (Atherley and Martin, 1971):

$$\text{ECNL} = 85{\cdot}4 + 20 \log_{10}(P_h) + 10 \log_{10}(n) + 10 \log_{10}(t_e) + 10 \log_{10}(1 - e^{-2/ten})$$

where P_h is the peak height in Newtons per square meter, n is the number of impacts in the train, and t_e is the decay time in seconds. The decay time is the time taken for the envelope to fall to $1/e$ of its maximum height. The point $1/e$ is equal $P_h - 8{\cdot}7$ dB.

Startle Due to Sonic Boom

D. N. MAY

Institute of Sound and Vibration Research,
University of Southampton, Southampton, England

Startle research at the Institute of Sound and Vibration Research was instituted as part of a large programme to establish the effects of the sonic boom on humans (Rice and May, 1969; May, 1970; Rice and Lilley 1969; Large and May, 1971) as well as structures. While a number of startle effects are under study, including that on sleep (Morgan and Rice, 1970; 1971) the main effort to date has been to investigate the rather dramatic hypothesis that the involuntary limb movement which forms the startle response will precipitate accidents to people in industry and elsewhere (Rice and May, 1969). Unfortunately for the researchers, though doubtless fortunately for everyone else, there have been ethical and practical problems about resolving the question through exposing workers to sonic booms or sonic boom simulations. While records have been studied of claims arising when sonic boom overflights do occur, and while a survey has been made of startle-induced accidents arising from other impulsive stimuli (Rice and May, 1969), most of the work has been performed in the laboratory.

The ISVR work in this area (May and Rice, 1969; 1971; May, 1971c) has paralleled valuable work performed by Woodhead (1969) at the Applied Psychology Unit of the Medical Research Council; by Lukas and Kryter (1968) at Stanford Research Institute; by Thackray and Touchstone at the Civil Aeromedical Institute of the Federal Aviation Administration (Thackray, 1965; Thackray and Touchstone, 1970); by Rylander *et al.* (1970) at the Swedish Department of Environmental Hygiene; and by Vlasak (1969) at the Czechoslovak Institute of Aviation Medicine. The stimuli used in these experiments are sometimes booms or tape-recorded booms, but are more usually pisto shots or noise bursts. The tasks are "psychological" ones; an example in use at the ISVR is shown in Fig. 1. Psychophysical methods are also used.

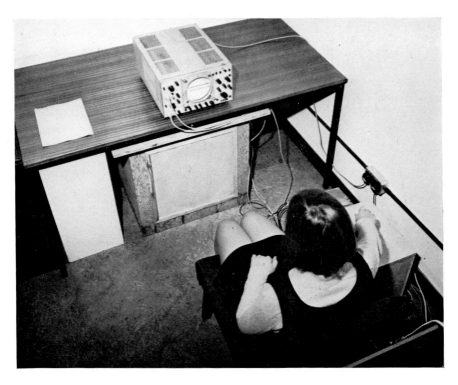

FIG. 1. Subject engaged on a single-axis pursuit tracking task to assess response to impulse
noise presented unexpectedly through the loudspeaker (see May, 1971c).

DURATION OF EFFECT

The duration of the startle response extends from about 40 millisec after
the stimulus to perhaps 500 millisec (Landis and Hunt, 1939), but the
direct consequences of the muscle flexure can be said to affect most
simple motor co-ordination tasks for about a further second (May and
Rice, 1969; 1971; Lukas and Kryter, 1968; Thackray, 1965; Thackray
and Touchstone, 1970; Vlasak, 1969).

Figure 2 shows a typical response in the seconds following a pistol
shot stimulus of subjects engaged on a pursuit rotor tracking task (May,
1970; May and Rice, 1971); the experimental group's scores are seen to
approach the control group's scores before three seconds had elapsed
after the stimulus presentation. However, more complex tasks, including mental ones, are affected for up to about half a minute (Woodhead,
1969; Vlasak, 1969), probably more through distraction than through
a spontaneous physiological mechanism.

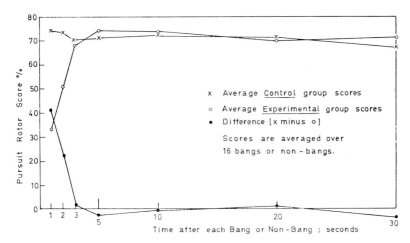

F ɪ ɢ . 2. Pursuit rotor performance following each bang (see May and Rice, 1971).

ADAPTATION AND EXPECTANCY

The rate of adaptation is generally regarded as being rather slow. Figure 3 shows the decrement in the amount of subjectively-measured startle induced in subjects during an experiment (May and Rice, 1969; 1971) in which they generally received one bang at a random moment in each of 20 three-minute sessions interspersed with two-minute rests.

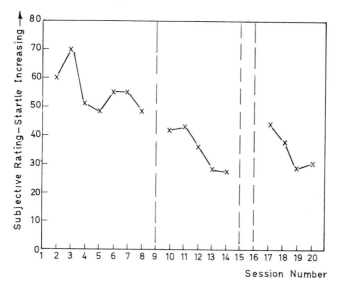

F ɪ ɢ . 3. Subjectively-rated startle as a function of number of presentations (see May and Rice, 1971).

Even after concentrated exposure like this, in a situation where they were obviously reasonably expectant, they remained startled at the end. A point of interest, however, is in the apparent "reversal of adaptation" which appeared after the long interval between presentations occasioned by the two consecutive stimulus-free sessions, 15 and 16.

This was tentatively explained by postulating a critical period after which subjects in a given situation lose their expectancy. In this experiment the period was a little over ten minutes. With more widely spaced sonic booms occurring in real life situations where people are unlikely to be able to concentrate on the prospect of the next stimulus, it is possible that startle reactions will not rapidly diminish with experience.

BACKGROUND NOISE

The effect of background noise on the startle response to a given boom might be expected to be such as to decrease the response—yet experiments with animals (Hoffman and Searle, 1968) produced contrary evidence. However an experiment with humans at the ISVR (May, 1971c) showed that the finding with animals did not extend to humans (see Fig. 4). Thus fears were somewhat allayed that workers in industrial

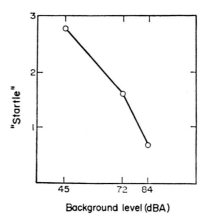

FIG. 4. Startle as a function of background level. Startle is defined as proportional to the increment in hand acceleration induced by an impulse in a subject engaged on a tracking task (see May, 1971c).

situations might be at risk not only because of the proximity of dangerous machinery, but also because of the presence of high levels of background noise.

EFFECTS OF STIMULUS PARAMETERS

The particular features in a pressure waveform which cause it to be startling are not clearly understood. Intensity is obviously one parameter, and Woodhead (1969) found significant impairment of performance at some levels of boom overpressure and not at others. Recent research at the ISVR has tried to separate the waveform parameters of importance by investigating correlations between startle judgements and various functions of the boom's overpressure and its rise time. These have yielded probably useful prediction equations for startle (May, 1971a), but it has not yet been shown that the functions governing startle are distinctly different from those governing loudness (May, 1971b).

DEPENDENCY ON PRE-STIMULUS PERFORMANCE

Two ISVR experiments have illustrated that the response is relatively independent of variables which normally affect task performance. Whereas performance is normally dependent on a subject's learning skill (i.e. "quicker learners achieve higher marks"), it was found (May and Rice, 1969; 1971) that performance during startle was independent of learning ability. In work not yet published, it has also been shown that the amplitude of the response is probably independent of the amplitude of the ongoing limb movement required to perform the task.

The preliminary inferences are that the response is not a function of many factors which generally govern task performance. Possibly, therefore, skilled workers are not protected from the effects of startle by virtue of their skill, and precision tasks are not protected from the effect of startle by virtue of their inherent intricacy. However there are too many unconsidered variables to safely extrapolate these findings to the operating theatre!

SUBGROUPS

Valuable early work by Landis and Hunt (1939) revealed subgroups of the population who exhibit abnormally large startle responses: schizophrenics, manic-depressives, and those who are feeble-minded or have hysteria. Woodhead (1969) showed that in a comparatively normal personality sample, people with tendencies towards neurosis exhibit larger responses. From commonsense reasoning it might be supposed that the anxious are especially susceptible to startle; but notwithstanding an early claim to the contrary (Large and May, 1971), a current ISVR study appears to indicate that there is not a significant correlation between the two.

No studies appear to have been carried out to determine whether the elderly or infirm are especially susceptible.

REFERENCES

Hoffman, H. S. and Searle, J. L. (1968). Acoustic and temporal factors in the evocation of startle. *J. acoust. Soc. Am.*, **43**, 2, 269.

Landis, G. and Hunt, W. A. (1939). "The Startle Pattern". Farrar and Rhinehart, New York.

Large, J. B. and May, D. N. (1971). U.K. research in sonic boom, SAE/DOT conference on aircraft and the environment, Washington DC, 8–10 February. *Paper* 710306.

Lukas, J. S. and Kryter, K. D. (1968). "Preliminary study of the awakening and startle effects of simulated sonic booms". *NASA CR*-1193.

May, D. N. (1970). Life with the boom. *Flight International*, **98**, Part I (1 October), p. 519; Part II (8 October), p. 563.

May, D. N. (1971a). Startle due to sonic booms heard outdoors as functions of overpressure and rise time. *J. Sound Vibrat.* **18**, 1, 144

May, D. N. (1971b). "The loudness of sonic booms heard outdoors as simple functions of overpressure and rise time". University of Southampton, Institute of Sound and Vibration Research, *Tech. Rep. TR* 46.

May, D. N. (1971c). Startle in the presence of background noise. *J. Sound Vibrat.*, **17**, **1**, 77.

May, D. N. and Rice, C. G. (1969). "Startle due to pistol shots: effects on control precision performance". University of Southampton Institute of Sound and Vibration Research, *Tech. Rep. TR* 26.

May, D. N. and Rice, C. G. (1971). Effects of startle due to pistol shots on control precision performance. *J. Sound Vibrat.*, **15**, **2**, 197.

Morgan, P. A. and Rice, C. G. (1970). "Behavioural awakening in response to indoor sonic booms". University of Southampton Institute of Sound and Vibration Research, *Tech. Rep. TR* 41.

Morgan, P. A. and Rice, C. G. (1971). "The effects of impulse noise on sleep— a behavioural awakening study". British Acoustical Society. Spring meeting, University of Birmingham, 5–7 April.

Rice, C. G. and Lilley, G. M. (1969). "Effects on humans (and animals) of the sonic boom". Part 4 of a report in five parts on the sonic boom, OECD conference on sonic boom research.

Rice, C. G. and May, D. N. (1969). "Startle due to sonic boom: statement of the problem". University of Southampton Institute of Sound and Vibration Research, *Tech. Rep. TR* 25.

Rylander, R., Sörensen, H., Berglund, H., Brodin, H. (1970). "Experiments on sonic boom exposure effects on humans". Paper presented at Acoustical Society of America second sonic boom symposium, Houston, Texas, 3 November.

Thackray, R. I. (1965). Correlates of reaction time to startle. *Human Factors*, **7**, 74.

Thackray, R. I. and Touchstone, R. M. (1970). Recovery of motor performance following startle. *Percept. Motor Skills*, **30**, 279.

Vlasak, M. (1969). Effect of startle stimuli on performance. *Aerospace Medicine*, **40**, **2**, 124.

Woodhead, M. M. (1969). Performing a visual task in the vicinity of reproduced sonic bangs. *J. Sound Vibrat.*, **9**, **1**, 121.

Some Personality Factors Influencing Hearing

S. D. G. STEPHENS*

M.R.C. Applied Psychology Unit, Cambridge,
and N.P.L., Teddington, England

Personality has been shown to influence many different aspects of hearing, and patients with certain auditory defects have been found to show distinctive changes in their personality. The general aspects of the influences of personality on hearing have been reviewed elsewhere, (Stephens, 1972), and can be classified under four main headings.

1. The effects on physiological responses to sound.
2. The effects on auditory perception.
3. The interaction with the effects of noise on performance.
4. The effects on noise annoyance.

The interactions of hearing loss and related clinical conditions with personality can likewise be subdivided into four main headings.

1. The personality changes found with specific disease entities.
2. The characteristic personality profiles found in patients with non-organic hearing loss (Chaiklin and Ventry, 1963; Trier and Levy, 1965).
3. Personality changes associated with profound deafness or deaf-mutism (Myklebust, 1964, Vernon, 1969, Remvig, 1969).
4. The differential effects of noise stress in precipitating psychological illness in patients with certain personality profiles.

In this paper I intend to consider how groups of personality variables may influence the results of a number of auditory measures, and how there can be an apparent change of personality in the course and treatment of certain disease entities.

A vast number of personality scales have been proposed and used at different times, but most of those used in relation to auditory studies can be considered as belonging to one of two groups of measures for which

* Now at ISVR, The University, Southampton.

173

a number of psychophysiological concomitants have been proposed. For convenience, I shall refer to these two groups as the "Introversion" group and the "Anxiety" group respectively.

"INTROVERSION" GROUP OF MEASURES

Perhaps the most fundamental group of personality variables are those which influence the psychological level of arousal, and hence the overall level of performance of the subject under different conditions. Many of these measures have been interrelated by a number of authors, and those which have been applied in auditory or other psychophysiological studies are shown in Table I.

TABLE I
"Introvert" Group

Weak	— Strong nervous system	(Teplov, 1964)
Augmentors	— Reducers	(Petrie *et al.*, 1963)
Receptives	— Non-receptives	(Reason, 1969)
Introverts	— Extraverts	(Jung, 1920; Eysenck, 1959)
Non-impulsives	— Impulsives	(Barratt, 1965)
Low Parmia	— High Parmia	(Cattell, 1965)
Ectomorphs	— Endomorphs/Mesomorphs	(Sheldon and Stevens, 1942)

Psychophysiological Concomitants

Salivation	(Corcoran, 1964)
Sedation threshold	(Shagass and Kerenyi, 1958)

Amongst these measures, Eysenck and Eysenck (1963) have shown that impulsiveness is one of the two main factors in their extraversion scale, the other being sociability. Parmia has been equated by Cattell (1965) with boldness or spontaneity.

In a rather different category are the somatotypes of Sheldon and Stevens (1942) and here the relationship is less direct. In their work they regard ectomorphs as being introverted and mesomorphs and endomorphs more extraverted. They found the ectomorphs were most sensitive to loud noises whereas mesomorphs, in particular, revelled in noisy conditions.

It must be emphasized at this stage that these various measures in this "Introvert" group are not assessing exactly the same factor and bear only a somewhat general relationship to each other. None is a perfect predictor of psychophysiological states, but such a predictor might conceivably be developed by extracting important factors from several of these approaches.

If these scales are attempting to assess the most basic of the personality factors, it is perhaps not surprising that they should have been applied in studies on the auditory threshold, which is probably the most fundamental of auditory measures. Nebylitsyn (1961) has endeavoured to relate the absolute sensitivity of the auditory threshold to the strength of the nervous system, subjects with a "weak" nervous system having more sensitive thresholds than those with a "strong" nervous system. Using somewhat complicated methodology, Smith (1968) has implicated the introversion-extraversion dimension in a similar way under certain circumstances. More orthodox audiometric and detection threshold techniques failed, however, to confirm any introvert-extravert differences in threshold sensitivity among larger groups of subjects (Stephens, 1969, 1971b).

The learning effects, or improvement in apparent sensitivity in threshold determinations on retesting, has been found by Delany (1970) to be frequency or order-dependent. For a group of audiometrically sophisticated subjects, introverts showed a greater learning effect than the extraverts (Stephens, 1971a).

Although the exact physiological origin of the auditory evoked response is unknown, it is by definition a physiological measure. In the context of somatosensory and visual evoked responses, Shagass and his associates (1965) have found a complicated relationship between extraversion and the amplitude of the evoked response. In a study on the auditory response Milner (1970) has found that, with long or irregular interstimulus intervals, the rate of growth of the evoked response amplitude with signal intensity above 70 dB sensation level is negatively related to their introversion.

In studies on auditory threshold variance, Robinson (1960) has proposed two major components originating from the subject, the variability of the absolute sensitivity, a somewhat physiological measure, and the variability of the response criterion, a more subjective measure. The relative contribution to the variance of these two measures can be separated by the use of techniques based on signal detection theory. The variability of the detection mechanism in these subjects has been related to their extraversion, extraverts showing larger variance than introverts, but the component of variance deriving from the response criterion is related to their neuroticism, neurotics showing greater variability than stable subjects (Stephens, 1969).

"ANXIETY" GROUP OF MEASURES

Neuroticism constitutes one of a second group of measures (Table II) to which I shall refer for convenience as the "anxiety" group. These are measures related to the "autonomic lability" of the subject and have been variously related to subjective aspects of hearing. The same limitations regarding their interrelationships and relative applicability apply to this group of measures as to the "introvert" group.

TABLE II
"Anxiety" Group

Neurotics	— Stables	(Eysenck, 1959)
Anxious	— Non-anxious	(Taylor, 1953; Cattell, 1965)
Test anxious	— Non test anxious	(Mandler and Sarason, 1952)
Failure avoidance motivated	— Non failure avoidance motivated	
		(Argyle and Robinson, 1962)
Low Ego-Strength	— High Ego Strength	(Dahlstrom and Welsh, 1960)

Psychophysiologcial Concomitants

Forearm blood-flow	(Kelly, 1966)
Finger-Pulse volume	(Ackner, 1956)
Electromyograms	(Malmo and Davis, 1951)
Sedation threshold	(Williams *et al.*, 1969)

With Békésy audiometry, the results obtained are more directly under the control of the subject and hence more susceptible to subjective factors. It is to be expected that they would be more influenced by the "anxiety" aspects of personality. It is therefore not surprising that Shepherd and Goldstein (1966, 1968) showed that the excursion amplitude in Békésy audiometry was related to the anxiety of the subject. Anxious subjects showed smaller excursion amplitude than less anxious subjects.

The assessment of loudness is again a very subjective exercise, and in two groups of subjects, the rate of increase of subjective loudness with physical intensity was found to be significantly related to the subject's test-anxiety score (Stephens, 1970a). Anxious subjects rated intense stimuli louder, and weak stimuli softer, than did the less anxious subjects.

Extending subjective loudness to audiometric practice, it is possible to consider its relevance to the uncomfortable loudness level (ULL). Using both a manual and semi-automatic (Békésy) presentation of the stimulus, the ULL was shown to be significantly negatively related to a measure of test-anxiety (Stephens, 1970b), so supporting the results of the loudness estimation study.

In both of the above experiments a varying relationship was found between the loudness measures and failure-avoidance motivation scores. The question therefore arises as to which scale in this "anxiety" group is the best predictor of subjects' susceptibility or otherwise to loud sounds. In a subsequent experiment, Fuller and Stephens (1971) administered neuroticism, test anxiety, failure-avoidance motivation scales and a manifest anxiety scale with three sub-scales (Fenz and Epstein, 1965) to a series of subjects. The test-anxiety scale was found to be the best predictor of both absolute ULL and also the ULL-most comfortable loudness level difference in this experiment.

From this account it may be seen that there is a certain amount of evidence to indicate that the "introversion" aspects of personality may influence the more "physiological" elements of auditory measures, and that the "anxiety" aspects may influence more the "subjective" elements.

PERSONALITY CHANGES IN THE COURSE OF AUDITORY DISORDERS

Hinchcliffe (1965, 1970), among others, has studied the personality changes in Ménière's disorder, and found a characteristic psychosomatic pattern on the Minnesota Multiphasic Personality Inventory (MMPI). In the course of these studies he showed that with increasing severity of the hearing loss, the deviation from normality in the triad of hysteria, hypochondriasis and depression become progressively less. This is in accord with the findings in other psychosomatic disorders such as hypertension (Davies, 1970), and has been interpreted as supporting the concept that the development of a psychosomatic condition is an alternative to the development of a neurosis or psychosis.

In his study, Hinchcliffe also found significantly increased neuroticism in his Ménière's disorder patients and also, more surprisingly, in his pre-operative otosclerotics. The question then arises as to whether this neuroticism is reduced when these patients undergo a successful stapedectomy. A recent study by Gildston and Gildston (1970) has gone far to providing an affirmative answer to this question. In their study they used the Guilford-Zimmerman personality scale which they administered to pre-operative otosclerotics, whom they showed to be significantly different from normal in a way that they could be regarded as being more neurotic and introverted. Two or three months after a successful stapedectomy they were retested and found to be significantly more normal, thus supporting the results presented by Ingham (1966) and others on psychiatric patients before and after treatment.

CONCLUSIONS

In this brief account I have endeavoured to show how two groups of personality variables may influence a number of audiometric measures.

I have also presented two examples which show that measures of a patient's personality may change during the course of an illness.

REFERENCES

Ackner, B. (1956). The relationship between anxiety and the level of peripheral vasomotor activity. *J. Psychosomat. Res.*, **1**, 21–48.

Argyle, M. and Robinson, P. (1962). Two origins of achievement motivation. *Brit. J. Soc. Clin. Psychol.*, **1**, 107–120.

Barratt, E. S. (1965). Factor analysis of some psychometric measures of impulsiveness and anxiety. *Psychol. Rep.*, **16**, 547–554.

Cattell, R. B. (1965). "The Scientific Analysis of Personality". Penguin Books, Harmondsworth.

Chaiklin, J. B. and Ventry, I. M. (1963). Functional hearing loss. *In* "Modern Developments in Audiology" (ed. J. Jerger), Academic Press, New York.

Corcoran, D. W. J. (1964). The relation between introversion and salivation. *Am. J. Psychol.*, **77**, 298–300.

Dahlstrom, W. G. and Welsh, G. S. (Eds) (1960). "An MMPI Handbook". University of Minnesota Press, Minneapolis.

Davies, M. (1960). Blood pressure and personality. *J. Psychosomat. Res.*, **14**, 89–104.

Delany, M. E. (1970). "On the Stability of Auditory Threshold". NPL Aero Report Ac., 44.

Eysenck, H. J. (1959). "Manual of the Maudsley Personality Inventory". University of London Press, London.

Eysenck, S. B. G. and Eysenck, H. J. (1963). On the dual nature of extraversion. *Brit. J. Soc. Clin. Psychol.*, **2**, 46–55.

Fenz, W. D. and Epstein, S. (1965). Manifest anxiety: unifactorial or multifactorial composition? *Percept. Motor Skills*, **20**, 773–780.

Fuller, H. and Stephens, S. D. G. (1971). (In prep.)

Gildston, H. and Gildston, P. (1970). "Personality Changes Associated with Surgically Corrected Hypacusis". Paper presented at 10th International Congress of Audiology, Dallas.

Hinchcliffe, R. (1965). A psychophysiological investigation into vertigo. Unpublished Ph.D. thesis, University of London.

Hinchcliffe, R. (1970). La maladie de Ménière. *Cahiers d'O.R.L.*, **5**, 725–732.

Ingham, J. G. (1966). Changes in MPI Scores in neurotic patients: a three-year follow-up. *Brit. J. Psychiat.*, **112**, 931–939.

Jung, C. G. (1924). "Psychological Types". (Transl. H. G. Baynes), Kegan Paul and Trubner, London.

Kelly, D. H. W. (1966). Measurement of anxiety by forearm bloodflow. *Brit. J. Psychiat.*, **112**, 789–798.

Malmo, R. B. and Davis, J. F. (1951). Electromyographic studies of muscular tension in psychiatric patients under stress. *J. clin. exp. Psychopath.*, **12**, 45–66.

Mandler, G. and Sarason, S. B. (1952). A study of anxiety and learning. *J. Abnorm. Soc. Psychol.*, **47**, 166–173.

Myklebust, H. R. (1964). "The Psychology of Deafness", 2nd ed. Grune and Stratton, New York.

Nebylitsyn, V. D. (1961). Individual differences in the strength and sensitivity of both visual and auditory analysers. *In* "Recent Soviet Psychology" (ed. N. O'Connor), Pergamon, Oxford.

Petrie, A., Holland, T. and Wolf, I. (1963). Sensory Stimulation Causing Subdued

Experience: audio-analgesic and perceptual augmentation and reduction. *J. Nerv. Ment. Dis.*, **137**, 312–321.

Reason, J. T. (1969). Individual differences in Motion Sickness Susceptibility: a further test of the "receptivity" hypothesis. *Brit. J. Psychol.*, **60**, 321–328.

Remvig, J. (1969). Three clinical studies on deaf-mutism and psychiatry. *Acta Psychiat. Scand.* Supp., **210**.

Robinson, D. W. (1960). Variability in the realization of the audiometric zero. *Ann. Occup. Hyg.*, **2**, 107–126.

Shagass, C. and Kerenyi, A. B. (1958). Neurophysiologic Studies of Personality. *J. Nerv. Ment. Dis.*, **126**, 141–147.

Shagass, C. and Schwartz, M. (1965). Age, personality and somatosensory cerebral evoked responses. *Science*, **148**, 1359–1361.

Shagass, C., Schwartz, M. and Krishnamoorti, S. R. (1965). Some psychological correlates of cerebral responses evoked by light flashes. *J. Psychosomat. Res.*, **9**, 223–231.

Sheldon, W. H. and Stevens, S. S. (1942). "The Varieties of Temperament". Harper and Bros., New York.

Shepherd, D. C. and Goldstein, R. (1966). Relation of Békésy tracings to personality and electrophysiologic measures. *J. Speech. Hear. Res.*, **9**, 385–411.

Shepherd, D. C. and Goldstein, R. (1968). Intrasubject variability in amplitude of Békésy tracings and its relation to measures of personality. *J. Speech Hear. Res.*, **11**, 523–535.

Smith, S. L. (1968). Extraversion and Sensory threshold. *Psychophysiology*, **5**, 293–299.

Stephens, S. D. G. (1969). Auditory threshold variance, signal detection theory, and personality. *Int. Audiol.*, **8**, 131–137.

Stephens, S. D. G. (1970a). Personality and the slope of loudness function. *Quart. J. exp. Psychol.*, **22**, 9–13.

Stephens, S. D. G. (1970b). Studies on the uncomfortable loudness level. *Sound*, **4**, 20–23.

Stephens, S. D. G. (1971a). Some individual factors influencing audiometric performance. *In* "Occupational Hearing Loss". (ed. D. W. Robinson), Academic Press, London.

Stephens, S. D. G. (1971b). The value of personality tests in relation to diagnostic problems of sensorineural hearing loss. *Sound*, **5**, 73–77.

Stephens, S. D. G. (1972). Hearing and personality: a review. *J. Sound Vib.* **20**, 287–297

Taylor, J. A. (1953). A personality scale of manifest anxiety. *J. Abnorm. Soc. Psychol.*, **48**, 285–290.

Teplov, B. M. (1964). Problems in the study of general types of higher nervous activity in man and animals. *In* "Pavlov's Typology" (ed. J. A. Gray), Pergamon, Oxford.

Trier, T. R. and Levy, R. (1965). Social and psychological characteristics of veterans with functional hearing loss. *J. Aud. Res.*, **5**, 241–256.

Vernon, M. (1969). Sociological and psychological factors associated with hearing loss. *J. Speech Hear. Res.*, **12**, 541–563.

Williams, J. G. L., Jones, J. R. and Williams, B. (1969). A physiological measure of preoperative anxiety. *Psychosomat. Med.*, **31**, 522–527.

Uses and Abuses of Speech Audiometry

R. R. A. COLES, A. MARKIDES
and VILIJA M. PRIEDE

Operational Acoustics and Audiology Group, Institute of Sound and Vibration Research, University of Southampton, Southampton, England

The potential advantages of speech audiometry are not widely appreciated in this country. In most of the places where it is carried out, either the technique is faulty or the results are wrongly interpreted, so much so, that the term "abuse" included in the title of this paper is justified. Our purpose, therefore, is to review the potential uses of speech audiometry and to comment on its abuses.

A brief outline of the nature of the technique and of the principal measurements derived from it will be given first. Lists of speech material, commonly phonetically-balanced (PB) monosyllabic words, are presented by live voice, loudspeaker or earphones at various levels of amplification and the percentage of the speech material correctly discriminated by the listener at each presentation level is then plotted on a graph—see the speech audiogram shown in Fig. 1.

One of the most commonly used terms in speech audiometry is the "speech reception threshold" (SRT). This measure usually refers to the sound level at which 50 per cent of spondee words (or some other percentage if other speech material is used, perhaps only 20 per cent for some PB word lists) are correctly discriminated. This in turn infers 100 per cent intelligibility for contextual speech; thus the term SRT is misused when applied to those cases of sensori-neural hearing loss in whom intelligibility of speech can never reach 100 per cent. Moreover, a rigid 50 per cent level, or 40 per cent as used by some, for defining SRT is unrealistic, as the speech discrimination of some cases of sensori-neural hearing loss never reaches 50 per cent, even for spondee words. Therefore, a better measurement and term is the half-peak level (HPL) which is the sound level at which the discrimination per cent is half that corresponding to the peak of the speech discrimination curve. Not only is the HPL a more practical measure in cases of severe sensori-neural

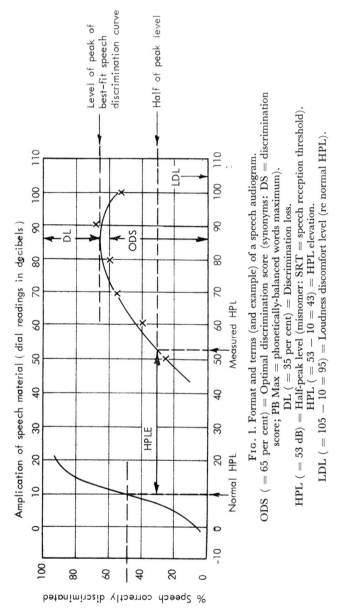

FIG. 1. Format and terms (and example) of a speech audiogram.

ODS (= 65 per cent) = Optimal discrimination score (synonyms: DS = discrimination score; PB Max = phonetically-balanced words maximum).

DL (= 35 per cent) = Discrimination loss.

HPL (= 53 dB) = Half-peak level (misnomer: SRT = speech reception threshold).

HPL (= 53 − 10 = 43) = HPL elevation.

LDL (= 105 − 10 = 95) = Loudness discomfort level (re normal HPL).

deafness, who never achieve a 100 per cent discrimination score, but it also correlates better with the "pure-tone-average" of those cases with sloping pure-tone audiograms. The "half-peak level elevation" (HPLE) refers to the difference between the pathological and the normal HPL.

The "optimal discrimination score", ODS, can be taken as the score corresponding to the highest point of the best-fit speech discrimination curve, but being an important measure more or less defined by a single point, it is really better to perform as precise a measurement as possible, using a relatively large amount of speech test material. For this we have up to now, used a whole Fry's PB word list, scored for each of its 100 phonemes.

Finally there is the LDL for speech. In our experience, this has little differential diagnostic significance, i.e. as a form of recruitment test to distinguish between sensory and neural types of auditory disorder. It provides, however, a useful guide regarding the tolerance threshold for speech of the patient, and this in turn is highly relevant to the selection and use of a hearing aid.

APPLICATIONS OF SPEECH AUDIOMETRY

The applications of speech audiometry can be placed into five main categories. This paper will be concerned with the first four only, together with one aspect which is common to all its applications: calibration.

TESTS OF AUDITORY ABILITY
General clinical assessment
Pre- and post-operative assessment
Auditory handicap assessment

AUDIOLOGICAL DIAGNOSIS
Sensori- vs. -neural dysfunction
Central deafness (by speeded, slowed, interrupted, filtered, monaural/binaural, speech)

DETECTION OF NON-ORGANIC HEARING LOSS
Speech vs. pure-tone thresholds
Atypical responses
Special forms (Doerfler-Stewart, delayed speech feedback, swinging voice, modified Stenger, dichotic filtered voice)

HEARING-AID ASSESSMENT
General information on the likely requirements (gain needed, usable intensity range, maximum output)
Trial of individual aids

Possible advantages of binaural fitting (squelch and
head-shadow advantages)

EXPERIMENTAL

Test of communication systems

Tests of effects of hearing protectors

Studies of effects of hearing-aid characteristics, e.g. frequency
response, tone controls, output limitation, distortion products.

CALIBRATION OF SPEECH AUDIOMETRY

The Ordinate : Per Cent Speech Correctly Discriminated

For any given intensity or level of amplification, the discrimination
score will depend to a crucial extent on a number of variables. These
must be defined before speech audiometric data can be quantified
meaningfully.

First, there is the speech material itself which ranges from relative
ease to relative difficulty, from sentences, through spondee or PB
words, to nonsense syllables, though even this is not an exhaustive list
as there are several other forms available, e.g. consonant-confusion
word lists. The most commonly used speech materials in Britain are
PB word lists, ranging from Fry's ten 35-word lists to Boothroyd's
fifteen 10-word lists.

Second, there is the quality of the speech. Governing this there is
the clarity and sex of the speaker's voice, accent, and the quality of
both the recording and the playback equipment, and the method of
recording (i.e. equal VU meter response, equal vocal effort, natural
intensity after a carrier-phrase of constant intensity). Any calibration
that is correct for one recording of a particular speech test material
cannot be taken to be correct for another.

It has been argued that hearing for both male and female voices
should be tested, as the majority of hard-of-hearing persons tend to
complain of greater difficulty in hearing female voices. This is true, but,
as will be explained when compensation assessment is discussed, it is
impossible to test all possible conditions and types of speech. Apart
from that, one would in the end obtain little more than multiple
measurements of the same thing. The speaker's accent will also affect
the results according to its familiarity to the listener, as indeed will be the
listener's own dialect, knowledge of the language, etc; but, with
the exception of some immigrant and foreign patients, the majority of
adults in this country are familiar with the relatively standard-English
accent and dialect of radio and television announcers. This is, therefore,
probably the best voice to utilize in recordings of speech test material.

Third, the method of scoring needs definition. With PB words, either the whole word or its constituent phonemes can be scored. In two subjective calibrations of our own clinical and experimental equipment and techniques, using persons with normal hearing and patients with conductive or perceptive deafness, the two scoring methods resulted in differences of 4 and 6 dB, phoneme scoring giving the more sensitive HPL values. The differences between phonemes and word scores will of course depend on whether the instructions given are specific for word or for phoneme scoring, the differences being greater with the instructions appropriate to phoneme scoring (the instructions used in our calibrations).

Any differences between word-scored and phoneme-scored results affect the ODS greatly, and conclusions dependent on the ODS can only be drawn from the particular speech material and recording, method of scoring and appropriate instructions. All these factors would also affect the HPL values. The scoring method and instructions would however have little effect on the HPLE because the per cent score used to derive the HPL of a pathological case depends on the height reached by the speech discrimination curve (obtained by the same method). This provides a further argument for using the HPL measurement rather than the 50 per cent level.

The ability of the tester is yet another variable, particularly in the case of phoneme scoring, but it is really impossible to have a separate calibration for each tester. Instead, one must resort to uniform and careful instruction of the patient and training of the tester, by which the former understands and performs the task properly and the latter instructs and scores properly. The instructions recently agreed for our own clinical use of speech audiometry, which are specific to phoneme scoring and should not be used for word scoring, are as follows:

> You are going to listen to someone speaking single words through the earphones. These words are spoken rhythmically like this . . . shop . . . bus . . . fun . . . toy. To start with, these words will be fairly loud but eventually I'll make them very quiet. Please listen carefully and repeat after each word whatever you think you heard. Even if you hear only part of the word, or a word that does not make sense or even a single sound like /a/, /o/ or /p/ please repeat whatever you heard because it adds to your score. Do you have any questions?

The Abscissa : Level (dB) of Amplification of Speech Material

The meaning of the decibel scale placed on speech audiometer attachments or speech facilities embodied in audiometers is most uncertain in this country at any rate, because there is no standard method for quantifying speech. Any physical calibration must take into account the time constant of the measuring equipment and the level quoted must refer to an agreed proportion of the words reaching that level when measured with the defined equipment: thus, a time/intensity distribution analysis is needed. The calibration tone should then bear some agreed relationship to this carefully quantified level of speech.

However good the physical calibration may be though, it cannot take account of all the variables listed in the previous subsection. Thus subjective calibration and proving is needed. Once this has been done, in one laboratory, it can be utilized elsewhere provided the same speech materials and recording (including its particular calibration tone), playback equipment, and methods are used.

This subjective calibration can best be achieved with a group of persons, whose thresholds of hearing in the test ear are within normal limits; say ten persons, with essentially flat pure-tone audiograms, in the -10 to $+20$ dB range, between 250 and 4,000 Hz. The pure-tone hearing level is averaged over 500, 1,000 and 2,000 Hz and between all ten test ears. Word lists are then presented at a suitable series of intensities, and the HPL is judged to the nearest 1 dB. The HPLs of all ten test ears are also averaged, and are then corrected for the average pure-tone level of the subjects employed. This provides the calibration of the speech audiometer in terms of the pure-tone audiometer. The pure-tone audiogram and HPL of any patient may then be compared quantitatively for diagnostic purposes, provided the same instruments and methods are used. Of course, if subsequently a different pure-tone audiometer is used with a different size of attenuator step (commonly 5 dB) or a different calibration, or if the audiometer's acoustic output alters, then corrections for change in attenuator-step size or in pure-tone calibration would have to be made to the relative calibration of the speech audiometer. (Note that considerable tolerances are allowed in audiometer calibration standards, and variations in acoustic output within the limits set by the standard can be too large to be acceptable for purposes of quantitative comparisons of pure-tone threshold and HPLE.)

In the case of Fry's tape recordings of his PB word lists, played from good quality (Ferrograph series 5) tape recorders, through Amplivox type 14950 speech audiometer attachments adjusted precisely to its manufacturer's specifications, to Telephonics TDH-39 ear-phones, and scored by phonemes heard correctly, we have made two independent calibration studies. The normal monaural HPL was at 4 dB nominal speech level (after correction had been made for minor deviations from zero pure-tone hearing level as measured with an audiometer using 5 dB attenuator steps, but not including corrections for the effect of the pure-tone attenuator step size).

In clinical practice, where to save time we have until recently used word-scoring (but with instructions appropriate to phoneme-scoring), and where we compare the HPLE with the pure-tone average obtained with 5 dB step audiometers, we have taken as our normal HPL a dial figure of 10 dB. It is this value that is shown as "normal" in Figs. 1, 3 and 4.

There is quite a wide (25 dB) range of variation in sensitivity between different types of audiometers and ear-phones used for speech audio-metry, and even within a given type or model. Therefore some expression of the acoustic output for a given setting of the speech dial is needed. With the equipment listed above, when the speech dial was set to 90 dB, the calibration tone from Fry's tape recordings gave a level of 117 dB in an IEC artificial ear (116 dB in a NBS 9A coupler). The normal HPL value of a 4 dB, reported above, should not be used, therefore, until the calibration of the complete equipment (from the calibration tone linked to the speech recording, through to the ear-phone output) has been checked and an appropriate correction factor applied to the 4 dB figure.

TESTS OF AUDITORY ABILITY

When considering the rehabilitation of a patient, and especially the educational management of a deaf child, it is very valuable to have a quantitative measure of ability to hear speech, not only at threshold but at suprathreshold levels as well. Unfortunately, this aspect of audiology tends to be overlooked, mainly because of the limitations of time, staff and equipment found in the majority of clinics.

Another important function of speech audiometry is for the testing of patients before and after stapedectomy and other surgical procedures in the ear. The point here is not so much to measure the reduction in degree of deafness, provided by the reduction in HPLE, which can easily be judged from the pure-tone audiogram, as to check on the degree to which this may be accompanied by a post-operative fall in ODS, i.e. the development or increase of a discrimination loss. This quite frequently occurs in those patients who exhibit a high-tone sensori-neural loss following operation. The patient may be satisfied with the operation in the sense that he can now hear sounds where previously they were too faint or he can now dispense with a hearing aid, but in constructive analysis of surgical results leading possibly to revision or refinements of technique it is as well to consider the debit part of the balance also, by means of ODS determinations. But in doing so, the need for careful masking is paramount; unfortunately this is particularly difficult in cases of conductive deafness, and masking problems quite often prohibit reliable speech audiometric measurements in such cases.

Perhaps the greatest spur towards more widespread adoption of speech audiometric tests in this country will come when industrial noise-induced hearing loss becomes compensatable under the National Insurance (Industrial Injuries) Act. If the recommendations of the British Association of Otolaryngologists are followed, both pure-tone threshold and speech-audiometric HPL and ODS measurements will be utilized in assessment of patients. These appear to have three potential merits: (i) as an indication of degree of handicap, (ii) in detection of non-organic hearing loss, which would then need more detailed investigation including objective audiometric tests and (iii) in differential diagnosis of sensory from neural types of disorder, noise deafness being sensory and potentially compensatable financially, neural lesions being not compensatable but the patient benefiting by their detection earlier than otherwise would have been the case. The second and third items will be discussed in later sections, but the first one belongs to this section.

A misconception is apt to creep in here. Because speech tests are more realistic than pure-tone ones and apparently more closely related to the handicap complained of, they tend to be regarded as better measures of the handicap itself. This may well be so, but there are three serious drawbacks.

The first drawback is that there are no really adequate speech audiometric tests which can be relied upon to *measure* the speech loss in individuals who are exaggerating their auditory impairment, as many do in cases seeking compensation (Coles and Priede, 1971). The Doerfler-Stewart and delayed speech feedback tests are only of real value in *detecting* some cases of non-organic hearing loss: for quantitative measurement of HPL they have grave limitations and they do nothing to verify the ODS. Claims have been made for cortical evoked response speech audiometry, but these do not really stand up to scientific criticism.

The second drawback is that it is impracticable in terms of test time and complexity to construct speech test materials which adequately reflect even a broad sample of the myriad variables of speech communication, such as the levels and quality of voices, levels, durations and spectra of background noise interference, degree of reverberation in the acoustic environment, that occur in everyday listening at home, at work, in travel, and in social life. If proper scientific standards are to be applied, as they must be, a single sample of voice, of speech material and of listening conditions has to be employed; and this involves a considerable loss of the realism ascribed to speech audiometry.

The third drawback is that there is surprisingly little evidence that auditory impairment measured by speech audiometry correlates with social handicap any better than do pure-tone audiometric measurements. The most recent study in this field is that of Acton (1971), working in collaboration with members of the Department of Social and Occupational Medicine in the University of Dundee (Kell *et al.*, 1971). He evaluated social handicap by means of a lengthy and searching questionnaire in 120 cases of industrial deafness, mostly weavers and boilermakers, together with various age-, status-, and dialect-matched control groups (N = 71 in all), and also obtained their pure-tone thresholds, their 50 per cent discrimination levels in quiet and in noise, and a form of ODS measurement in quiet and in noise. The best correlation (−0·70) between handicap and measurement was with the control-corrected arcsin-transformed noise-masked ODS, but for reasons beyond the scope of this paper this measure would be very difficult to administer for compensation assessment.

The next highest correlations (0·63 to 0·66) came from various combinations of pure-tone threshold, of which the 1,000, 2,000 and 3,000 Hz average would be the best combination of high correlation and practicability. His various 50 per cent discrimination measures, in quiet or in noise, gave correlations with handicap ranging from 0·49 to 0·52 only. Interestingly, the best correlation between any of the measurements with each other or with handicap was that (0·85) between the 50 per cent discrimination level in quiet and the 500, 1,000 and 2,000 Hz average; on the other hand, the 500, 1,000, 2,000 Hz average correlated relatively poorly (0·57) with social handicap, but still slightly better than did the 50 per cent discrimination level.

In short, the 1,000, 2,000 and 3,000 Hz average gave the best practical correlation with handicap, whilst the 500, 1,000 and 2,000 Hz average was a good predictor of the 50 per cent discrimination level in quiet. None of the other practicable speech audiometric measurements was nearly such a good index of social handicap as the 1,000, 2,000 and 3,000 Hz average. Thus, according to both Acton's study and earlier ones, speech audiometry would seem to have little or no advantage over pure-tone tests for purposes of assessment for compensation purposes of the *degree* of disability arising from industrial hearing loss. It will, however, in combination with clinical and other audiological observations, help towards an overall evaluation of the patient's handicap.

AUDIOLOGICAL DIAGNOSIS

Developments of speech audiometry may well come to find extensive uses in connection with tests designed to detect and locate lesions of the auditory tracts and their connections within the central nervous system.

However, these tests have not yet been developed sufficiently to be widely applicable in clinical work. In the meantime, conventional speech audiometry has much to offer at the peripheral and psychic ends of the auditory system.

Tests of sensori-neural hearing loss in fact distinguish between sensory and peripheral neural *patterns* of *dysfunction*, rather than between cochlear and retrocochlear *sites of lesion*, as has been pointed out recently by one of us (Coles, 1971). However, time factors tend to limit the extent of the audiological investigation that can be carried out and a form of "diagnostic strategy" becomes necessary. In this, the tests available for sensori-neural hearing loss have been classified (Coles and Priede, 1973a) into three types according to the way in which they test some particular function or dysfunction, thus:

Tests of loudness recruitment, e.g. alternate binaural loudness balance (Fowler), acoustic reflex threshold (Metz)

Tests of abnormal adaptation, e.g. tone decay (Carhart, Owens), Békésy, audiometry (Jerger)

Tests of abnormal discrimination, e.g. of speech, or of small pure-tone intensity changes (Jerger, Shedd and Harford's SISI test, Luscher and Zwislocki's difference limen test)

Where time is very limited and the hearing loss pattern is suitable i.e. sensori-neural loss is unilateral, the ABLB test is probably the best. But its results are often equivocal, and sometimes misleading unless one recalls that disease of and around the VIIIth cranial nerve can result in secondary damage to the sensory elements in the cochlea with the complete recruitment typical of hair-cell damage and that sensory lesions often lead to secondary neural degeneration with consequent lack of complete recruitment. Other recruitment tests would, by and large, yield the same results. It is better therefore to perform one test from each of the above groups rather than several tests from one group; quite often, neural degrees of adaptation and discrimination loss are found to accompany complete recruitment, and thereby give due warning that the primary site of lesion may not be wholly cochlear after all. In our opinion, of the tests available, the ODS determination ranks at least as equal in reliability to the ABLB test and greater in range of applicability, in that it is not restricted to unilateral cases.

Some aspects of the differential diagnostic value of speech audiometry is subject to studies by one of us (VMP). The final results are not yet complete, but a preliminary analysis* is shown in Fig. 2. This

* The analysis is currently being extended, and also modified in respect of the pure-tone-average formula for rising audiometric configurations and of corrections for word list differences, and the results shown in Fig. 2 are only preliminary. For Fry's word lists and phoneme scoring, they already have considerable diagnostic value however, and may be used, with discretion, in their present state provided the tape recorder, attenuator and earphone are of good quality; if poor, or if free-field conditions, the "criteria" will probably be quite different.

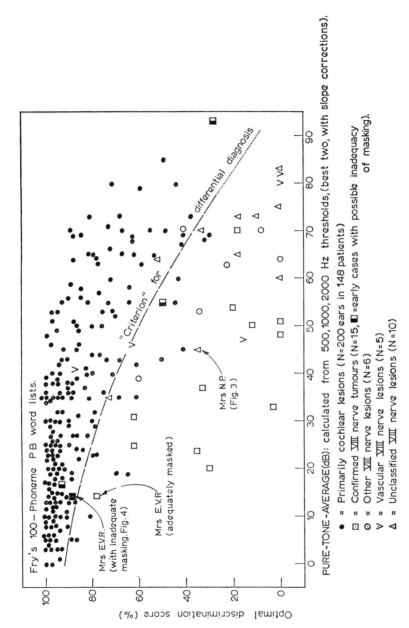

FIG. 2. Optimal speech discrimination as a test for differentiating sensory from neural hearing loss.

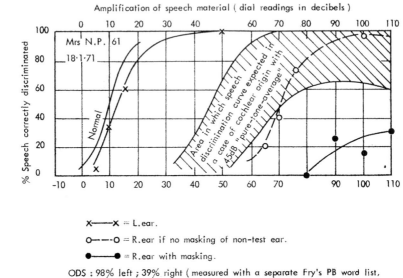

Amplification of speech material (dial readings in decibels)

x——x = L.ear.

o———o = R.ear if no masking of non-test ear.

●———● = R.ear with masking.

ODS : 98% left ; 39% right (measured with a separate Fry's PB word list, with masking of non-test ear).

HPLE : 13 – 10 = 3dB left ; 88 – 10 = 78 dB right.

FIG. 3. Speech audiogram of a neural case, with and without masking.

shows the ODS results as a function of the pure-tone-average* hearing losses of 184 patients with sensori-neural hearing losses of acquired type. As might be expected, the ODS values of the cases with primarily cochlear lesions were generally higher than those of patients with neural lesions. The "criterion" line drawn by eye between the two types of patient separates the two to an accuracy which compares well with other test techniques, e.g. ABLB, about 90 per cent of the cochlear lesions having ODS values above the line and a similar proportion of the neural cases being below the line.

It is pointed out, however, that abnormally low scores do not necessarily relate solely to neural patterns of dysfunction. Some patients with steeply falling pure-tone audiogram configurations, senile patients suffering from phonemic regression, people with severe articulation problems, patients who experience difficulties in understanding the spoken word and people who have either defective memory or limited attention span might also produce disproportionately low speech discrimination scores.

*The averaging formula used here was to average the best two of the three frequencies, 500, 1,000, 2,000 Hz and to add a factor according to slope of the audiogram: thus, if the hearing level at 4,000 Hz is 11–20 dB greater than the BTA then 1 dB was added, if 21–30 dB greater 2 dB was added, if 31–40 dB greater 3 dB was added, if over 40 dB greater 4 dB was added.

Somewhat similar differential-diagnostic results may well result from analyses of HPL measurements (see Fig. 5, discussed in the next section). Occasionally, the speech discrimination of a patient with a peripheral neural lesion may be within those expected of a sensory lesion at the optimal level, but be quite abnormal at lower and/or higher levels. Suffice to say at the present that it is advisable to plot the whole speech discrimination curve as well as measure the ODS.

The diagnostic value of speech audiometric measurements, together with possible pitfalls in technique, are illustrated by two examples. In Fig. 3 is shown the speech audiogram of a case with a unilateral neural type of hearing loss. The true discrimination curve of the right ear, when the left ear was properly masked, is that drawn through the data points plotted with the closed circle symbol. The shaded area represents the area in which the discrimination curve would be expected if proportional to the pure-tone audiogram, i.e. a sensory type of hearing loss. The data points marked with the open circle symbol were the right-ear results obtained when no masking had been applied to the non-test ear; they were simply a shadow of the left ear. The message is simple. Without masking of the non-test ear, the speech tests suggested a sensory type of dsyfunction; with appropriate masking, they suggested the true state of affairs—a neural lesion.

The second, more recent, example is shown in Fig. 4. Although this woman had a pure-tone audiogram that was virtually normal, she had a number of alerting symptoms suggestive of a neural lesion, notably a numbness of the left side of the face and a dullness of sounds when she put a telephone to her left ear. Her normal audiogram was therefore

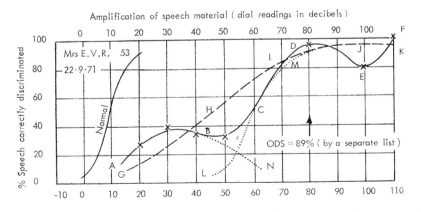

F I G. 4. Speech audiogram of a neural case, inadequately masked.

not accepted as conclusive evidence of normality. Further tests showed in the left ear a marked tone decay, loudness reversal, partial canal paresis, and the speech audiogram depicted. She had, in fact, a left acoustic neuroma, successfully removed soon afterwards.

The speech discrimination curve ABCDEF had a curious wavelike configuration, known to occur in patients with a high-frequency plateau in their pure-tone audiogram. However this could not have been the explanation in this case, as there was no appreciable high-frequency hearing loss. Instead, we were inclined at first to interpret the crests and troughs of her speech audiogram as being due to unusually erratic responses. The smoothed speech discrimination function GHIJK was postulated. The ODS was around the lower limit to be expected of persons with a normal pure-tone audiogram and without an incipient neural lesion: on the other hand, the HPLE was about 34 dB, which was certainly not to be expected from a normal ear.

Several further tests were performed next day, and her speech audiogram repeated, as some doubt existed as to the adequacy of the masking that had primarily been delivered to the non-test ear. A speech discrimination curve was obtained that had the general shape ABN but reaching to a higher level than before and accompanied by an ODS determination at 30 dB dial level of 78 per cent, which was more clearly diagnostic of a neural lesion (see Fig. 2). The apparent improvement at low speech intensities was attributed to a real change in auditory ability, as is known to occur sometimes over a short period of time in neural types of disorder.

The true interpretation of the original speech audiogram ABCDEF was now apparent. The masking had indeed been inadequate. Component AB was a correct measure of the speech discrimination ability of the left ear at low levels of amplification; but, instead of falling below point B, it merged into the shadow audiogram derived from the right ear, depicted as component LCM. The remainder of the smoothed curve, from I to M, through J, to K, was probably a correct smoothing of the original inadequately-masked data.

Techniques for masking of the non-test ear in speech audiometry are complicated, if proper account is to be taken of the many variables. Lidén et al. (1959) have provided a formula which takes account of some of the factors concerned, but two of us have recently* prepared a more comprehensive treatment of the subject (Coles and Priede, 1972b). The need for great care in masking in speech tests of hearing is illus-

---

* Until published, a "cookbook" set of formulae for calculation of how much masking is needed, the masking dial settings for use if masking is needed, and the extent of possible cross-masking that may occur, has been used for teaching purposes. Copies are available on application to the authors.

trated by the case of Mrs E.V.R. (Fig. 2), and by the three cases marked by the half-closed, half-open rectangle symbol in Fig. 2, where in spite of our special interest and awareness of the problem we have not always masked adequately. It may well be that the lack of general recognition of speech audiometry as perhaps the most potentially valuable of all tests for distinguishing between sensory and peripheral neural types of auditory dysfunctions is due to the poor results obtained as a result of inadequate masking of the non-test ear.*

DETECTION OF NON-ORGANIC HEARING LOSS

Apart from unilateral, and to some extent asymmetrical, cases, when the Stenger test has paramount value, speech audiometry offers the best test for detection of the presence of a significant non-organic element in an apparent hearing loss (Coles and Priede, 1971). Firstly, there are characteristic patterns of response which the experienced operator will learn to recognize; typical of these are responses in which the first or always the second consonant sound are wrong, responses regularly restricted to every second or third word, responses frequently with alternatives e.g. for the stimulus word "but" he might respond "but or cut", for "hid" respond "hid or head", etc., inconsistent (greater than ± 15 per cent) responses when the particular presentation level is repeated, or gross changes of discrimination score with only 5 dB change in presentation level, e.g. from over 80 per cent to under 20 per cent which are not compatible with even the steepest part (commonly 6 per cent per dB) of a PB-word discrimination curve. Since that publication, the authors have added a further 45 cases of non-organic hearing loss to their previous series of 70; 89 of these patients were tested with speech audiometry and 40 of them exhibited response patterns suggestive of non-organic loss.

The relationship between pure-tone thresholds and HPLE determinations is even more revealing with such patients. In our 89 non-organic cases tested with speech audiometry, 76 gave HPLE values that were inconsistent with the average of the best-two hearing levels at 500, 1,000 and 2,000 Hz; that is, there was more than a 10 dB discrepancy. In 74 of the 76, the HPLE's were more than 10 dB lower than indicated by the pure-tone thresholds, and in 34 of these 74, the HPLE's were either within normal values or within 11 dB of the true thresholds as estimated by such objective techniques as electrodermal, cortical evoked response or delayed tone feedback audiometry. Taking the evidence from both pattern of response and from consistency with

* Free-field test conditions have been used for speech audiometry in some clinics, but the range of masking levels between too little or too much is much narrower in this condition and is even more difficult to define.

o

the pure-tone audiogram, speech audiometry gave an indication or proof of non-organic hearing loss in no fewer than 84 of the 89 cases tested.

One must, however, examine also the correlations between pure-tone and speech audiometry that occur in cases of organic hearing loss. We have analysed these in 448 ears of 301 persons with normal hearing, or sensory types of hearing loss of acquired type.

The median HPL's for Fry's PB word lists, scored by phonemes and corrected for the pure-tone hearing levels (measured in 5 dB steps but not including corrections for the pure-tone audiometer's 5 dB step size) and for variations in the scoring methods actually used in individuals, were as follows in various groups of ears:

   (i) 197 ears with flat pure-tone audiometric
       configurations   ..   ..   3·8 dB
  (ii) 85 ears in which the 4,000 Hz threshold
       was 11–20 dB poorer   ..   ..   5·0 dB
 (iii) 63 ears in which the 4,000 Hz threshold
       was 21–30 dB poorer   ..   ..   5·5 dB
  (iv) 31 ears in which the 4,000 Hz threshold
       was 31–40 dB poorer   ..   ..   6·6 dB
  (v) 39 ears in which the 4,000 Hz threshold
       was over 40 dB poorer ..   ..   8·0 dB

Being "poorer" refers to the "best-two-average", i.e. the average of the two more acute thresholds in the 500, 1,000 and 2,000 Hz range, which would give the best correlation with hearing loss for speech according to the analyses of Fletcher (1950): indeed, the figures above are gratifyingly close to the 0 to +4 dB corrections to the best-two-average which Fletcher recommends in cases of high-tone hearing loss. Accordingly, in comparing HPLE and pure-tone threshold in an individual ear, we now add 0, 1, 2, 3 or 4 dB to the best two-average depending on whether the case fits into categories (i)–(v) respectively.

Thirty-three ears had rising audiometric configurations, seven of them steeply. Those having 500 Hz thresholds 11–20 dB poorer than the best-two-avearge required a correction factor of +3 dB, and those 21–30 dB poorer a correction factor of +10 dB.

Apart from these corrections for a slope of audiogram, the correlations between speech and pure-tone results were studied as a function of degree of hearing loss—310 had best-two-average values of between −10 and +30 dB, 99 between 31 and 60 dB, 39 of over 60 dB. The degree of hearing loss appeared to have no appreciable average effect on the good agreement between the best-two-average and HPLE.

The variability of the agreement between the best-two-average and

HPLE of individual cases is of course important whenever this is to be considered as a diagnostic tool. In fact, the range that we use clinically, i.e. ± 10 dB, covered 70–90 per cent of the ears tested, the poorer correlations relating to the ears with greater and/or steeper hearing losses.

Thus, comparison of pure-tone threshold and HPLE gives a good differentiation, to perhaps 80 per cent reliability using ± 10 dB tolerances, between non-organic and sensory hearing loss. On the other hand, the pure-tone and ODS comparison (Fig. 2) gives a similar or even better reliability for distinguishing between sensory and peripheral neural lesions. Probably, a similar sort of result will come from analyses, not yet complete, of our data comparing HPLE with the pure-tone threshold in sensory and peripheral neural cases. If so, one will be able to construct a graphical set of criteria of the type outlined in Fig. 5.

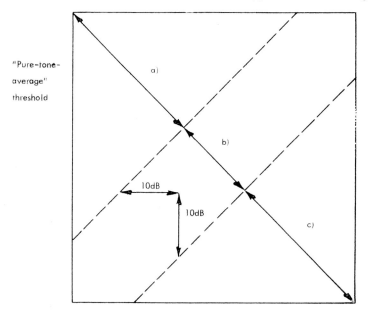

Half-peak level elevation (speech)

Fig. 5. Expected relationships between speech (HPLE) and pure-tone threshold: (a) Majority of cases of non-organic hearing loss. (b) Majority of cases of conductive or sensory hearing loss. (c) Majority of cases of peripheral neural hearing loss.

The concept of this figure provides a useful summary of the potential applications of speech audiometry in the diagnostic and compensation fields of audiology. In compensation work in particular, if the pure-tone threshold (best-two-average with slope corrections) and the HPLE do not agree to within ± 10 dB, then there may well be either a non-organic or peripheral neural type of hearing loss. If the HPLE is better, objective techniques available for pure-tone tests should be applied whenever possible; when not possible, the HPLE should at least be taken as the more reliable (in that case) indicator of the true auditory handicap. If the HPLE is worse, the case is potentially one of a more serious nature and demands full investigation for clinical purposes, as well as for compensation assessment purposes; indeed, if found to be of neural type, the hearing loss would not be due to a compensatable (noise-induced) disorder.

HEARING-AID ASSESSMENT

A straightforward speech audiogram of each ear separately, as shown in Fig. 1, can be most helpful in general assessment of a patient's hearing-aid requirement and of the limitations likely to be encountered. The HPLE and DL give indications of the degree of handicap of the patient. The ODS gives an idea of the maximum discrimination likely to be achieved from that ear when hearing-aided and the level at which such discrimination will occur. More usually though, an aid, being of "low-fidelity", gives somewhat poorer discrimination than indicated by the ODS; but in some instances, e.g. by vented earmoulds in case of gradual high-tone hearing loss, an aid can produce a more desirable frequency-weighting of the speech input which can give higher discrimination scores than indicated by the ODS. The LDL gives an indication of the upper limit of the patient's auditory range, and the possible need for a form of output limitation in a hearing aid for that patient.

So far, so good: speech audiometry can find worthwhile usage in connection with hearing-aid prescription. The seemingly obvious next step is to try out a selection of aids using speech as a test material for discrimination tests to help decide which aid best suits the particular patient. In this, there are two major potentialities for abuse.

Firstly, as with its use for quantifying an auditory handicap, it is not practicable to use a sufficient range of speech materials, listening conditions, competing noises, etc., to be fully representative of everyday life. The materials required would be far too lengthy for clinical usage. Quite apart from the great difficulty of preparing satisfactory sets of speech material for each aid to be tested, each set having to be statistically validated as being equally difficult, the test time involved would induce loss of precision due to mental fatigue effects. If the materials are then so restricted as to be practicable in a clinic, they are no longer fully representative of patients' communication environments. The abuse occurs when tests using conventional speech audiometric material are interpreted as anything more than an indicator (as distinct from a measure) of the patient's aided ability in everyday life.

The second comes from taking the speech audiometric results at their numerical face value. There are three main variables to consider.

(i) *Inequality of the word lists.* Various sets of word lists are available for speech audiometry but in few, if any, of them are the word lists (within one set) of equal difficulty. Correction factors, of up to about 10 per cent, have been worked out in some instances, but are not widely published let alone used. (Data on some of Fry's lists as applied to patients with sensori-neural hearing losses are being analysed by two of us, by AM in the case of free-field tests in quiet and in various levels of background noise and by VMP in the case of ear-phone tests in quiet, and will be published in due course.)

(ii) *Variability due to initial technique-learning and later mental-fatigue effects.* A trial list, which may have to be discarded, is needed to counteract the former effect and limited duration (perhaps 30 min.) of non-stop speech audiometric testing is needed to avoid the latter.

(iii) *Test/retest variance.* This varies between patients, some being good listeners and others poor. It is also of course highly dependent on the amount of speech material utilized to obtain the data by which the effectiveness of different hearing aids is to be compared and by which the intra-subject reliability of the patient may be measured. Frequently, it is too little, e.g. one 20-word list scored by words at the optimal level; on other occasions it could be too much, e.g. when a whole curve is plotted out with long word lists for each of a series of hearing aids or when the greater statistical reliability is counteracted by fatigue effects and time factors in the clinic make it hardly acceptable anyway. Taking the former case, of too little speech test material, Ewertsen (1967) using 25-word lists scored by words estimates the reliability of any one measurement as ± 12 per cent; Boothroyd (1968) using 10-word lists estimates the 95 per cent confidence limits of a single, near threshold (i.e. around 50 per cent score), phoneme discrimination measurement as ± 20 per cent. Allowing for the greater amount of test material, and correcting for inequalities between lists, we have estimated that the corresponding (95 per cent) reliability of one of Fry's 35-word PB word lists, scored by phonemes, would be about ± 10 per cent; this corresponds to a standard deviation of 5 per cent.

It is salutory to examine just what this means in practice, if free-field speech audiometric tests are used for hearing-aid selection. Take the situation where either aid A, aid B, or aid C would seem to suit a particular patient, and an attempt is made to measure the speech discrimination effectiveness of each aid in turn by presenting one 100-phoneme-word list at conversational voice level with the aid's gain set by the patient to the level that seems optimal in terms of clarity, loudness and comfort. What magnitude of difference in speech discrimination score measured by a single list can be regarded as a reliable indication of superiority, under these particular test conditions?

Assume for the moment that the patient is an average listener, i.e. that his particular test/retest standard deviation for repeated discrimination measurements with equally-difficult 100-phoneme-word lists is the 5 per cent already mentioned. One can then calculate the probability of whether an apparent difference in speech discrimination resulting when two successive hearing aids are worn might be a true expression of their rank-order merit. The results of such calculations are given in Table I below:

TABLE I

Difference in speech discrimination score	Chance that this is not a true rank-order representation of merit
18 per cent	1 in 100
16 per cent	2 in 100
14 per cent	5 in 100
12 per cent	9 in 100
10 per cent	16 in 100
8 per cent	26 in 100
6 per cent	40 in 100
5 per cent	48 in 100

In other words, for the particular speech condition/aids/patient, for a nine out of ten probability that the measurement means what it appears to mean, the difference in discrimination scores between the two aids would have to be 12 per cent or more. A two out of three probability requires a difference of 7 per cent or more. Whilst if the difference is less than 5 per cent, the chances are even as to which aid really performs best for the particular patient and test condition.

The trouble is that one is not using the test to compare aids which have grossly different performances, or at least one should not be if one is making a reasonable selection of possible aids. Instead, the true range of speech discrimination effectiveness, as measured by the speech discrimination tests exampled, in a group of three potentially suitable aids would probably not be greater than 10 per cent. Speech audiometry in quiet, is thus a blunt and unwieldy tool with which to test out these differences in individuals. However, if conducted in a background of noise, the performance differences between aids become more clearly defined. Speech tests in a competing noise background therefore have much greater potential value for testing an individual's hearing-aid needs.

There are further limitations on the above reliability assessments and the interpretations that can be drawn. The patient may not try so hard with an aid whose appearance, cost, etc., he may not like. Different word lists used for testing each aid may need to have correction factors (of up to 10 per cent) applied, if these factors are known. The length of the lists used may be considerably less than 100 phonemes, when the difference in scores between aids must be greater to achieve the same level of significance. The standard deviation of 5 per cent was a hypothetical estimate for the average listener, but some patients are more precise and others less so; whilst it is quite possible to measure the speech-audiometric reliability of a particular listener, this is not a very practicable procedure in a clinical setting. The tests and interpretations quoted only apply to comparisons of discrimination score where one of the scores is in the 20 per cent to 80 per cent region; if smaller word lists were used, then the discrimination per cent range of applicability of this technique would be narrower still. Finally, if the results of the test indicated that one particular aid was better than another, this assessment might not apply for conditions other than listening to clearly enunciated words, at conversational voice level, in a quiet background, in a room without high levels of reverberation, and with the aid of around optimal gain setting for these conditions. The test may well be an indication of its performance under a much wider range of conditions than the test ones listed above, but it is not necessarily so.

Speech tests can be used to back up the patient's assessment and the prescriber's experience and judgement, or to provide a casting vote when the balance of other considerations is equal, but it is an abuse of speech audiometry to place greater reliance on the results than that appropriate to the test materials and technique employed and to fail to take into account the many other factors discussed above.

There is however one further use for speech audiometry in hearing-aid assessment which appears more promising. This is in the testing of an individual's needs for binaural fitting of aids or restoration of binaural hearing advantages in a patient with unilateral deafness. A lengthy study by one of us (AM) on this subject is nearing completion now, and it is anticipated that it will lead to general rules based on knowledge of the patient's pure-tone audiogram and of the general type of disorder, e.g. conductive, sensory or neural, whereby the potential benefits of attempts at prosthetic restoration of binaural hearing can be judged. This is especially important in children for whom speech audiometric and other hearing-aid selection procedures would often be inappropriate. But in those adults and older children who have sufficient linguistic ability, it seems probable that judgements based on the rules to be defined can usefully be checked by clinical tests in individuals; we are already conducting such tests and the technique developed seems to be valuable.

ACKNOWLEDGEMENTS

The authors are indebted to many persons in helping with this paper, but notably Miss H. M. Ballam who searched countless audiological files both here and at the neuro-otology clinic at the Wessex Neurological Centre for all relevant speech-audiometric data, and Mr W. I. Acton for information on his pure-tone/speech/social handicap analyses. Different components of the work were supported in turn by the Medical Research Council (grant number 970/512/C), the Wates Foundation, and the Wessex Regional Hospital Board.

REFERENCES

Acton, W. I. (1971). Personal communication.

Boothroyd, A. (1968). Developments in speech audiometry. *Sound*, **2**, 3–10.

Coles, R. R. A. (1972). Can present day audiology really help in diagnosis?—An otologist's question. *J. Laryngol. Otol.*, **86**, 191–224.

Coles, R. R. A. and Priede, V. M. (1971). Non-organic overlay in noise-induced hearing loss. *Proc. R. Soc. Med.*, **64**, 194–199.

Coles, R. R. A. and Priede, V. M. (1973a). Diagnostic strategy. (In preparation.)

Coles, R. R. A. and Priede, V. M. (1973b). Masking of the non-test ear in speech audiometry. (In preparation.)

Ewertsen, W. H. (1967). Theoretical considerations and practical experience in hearing aid selection. *Sound*, **1**, 92–97.

Fletcher, H. (1950). A method of calculating hearing loss for speech from an audiogram. *J. acoust. Soc. Am.*, **22**, 1–5.

Fry, D. B. (1961). Word and sentence tests for use in speech audiometry. *Lancet*, ii, 197–199.

Kell, R. L., Pearson, J. C. G., Acton, W. I. and Taylor, W. (1971). Social effects of hearing loss due to weaving noise. *In* "Occupational Hearing Loss" (ed. D. W. Robinson), Academic Press, London.

Lidén, G., Nilsson, G. and Anderson, H. (1959). Masking in clinical audiometry. *Acta Oto-laryngol. Stockh.*, **50**, 125–136.

Some Applications of the Electro-Acoustic Analysis of Speech

J. J. KNIGHT

*Institute of Laryngology and Otology, University of London,
London, England*

Much progress in Audiology has resulted from collaboration between otolaryngologists and physicists in applying acoustic measuring techniques to hearing problems. There exists another field for similar collaboration in the application of acoustic techniques to the identification and specification of the physical characteristics of disordered speech which results from many pathological conditions.

INSTRUMENTATION AND METHODS

The acoustic properties of normal speech were studied 50 years ago by telephone engineers from waveforms, and the introduction of the speech spectrograph 25 years ago has added tremendously to the knowledge of phoneticians and others concerned with the analysis, and with the synthesis, of speech. The conventional speech spectrogram is a record of a passage of speech showing variations of intensity as patterns of light and shade on a graph with axes representing frequency content and time. In this record, the formants of speech produced by resonant excitation of the vocal cavities by the complex wave which originates from the vocal cords, are seen as a series of dark bars as in Fig. 1. Hence it has been called a "bar spectrogram". Lately, introduction of an amplitude quantizer for speech spectrographs has led to "contour spectrograms" in which a series of contours covering up to a 48 dB range are displayed at 6 dB intervals of intensity to aid visualization of speech patterns. Figure 2 shows a bar and a contour spectrogram of a male voice uttering the word "you".

In some applications, interest centres on intonation and on the regularity of the vocal cord vibration. This vibration has been examined by application of a contact microphone (von Leden and Koike, 1970), or an accelerometer, to the larynx. Ultrasonics and high frequency electrical

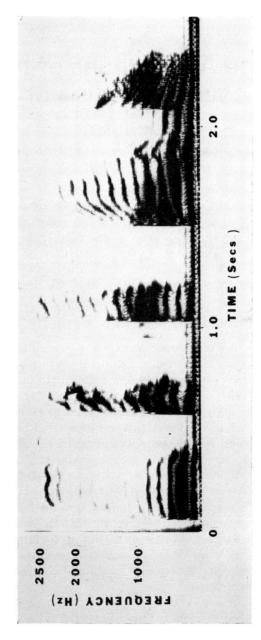

FIG. 1. Normal male voice. Spectrogram of "We sat up all night".

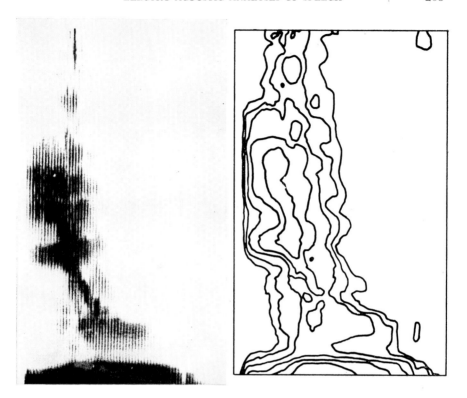

FIG. 2. Normal male voice. (a) Bar spectrogram of "you". (b) Contour spectrogram of "you".

sources have also been used to determine the movement of vocal cords; one of the most promising instruments using the latter method for detection of the resulting impedance changes across the vocal cords being the laryngograph recently described by Fourcin and Abberton (1971).

Statistical measurements have been applied to vocal spectra of individual voices by Bordone-Sacerdote and Sacerdote (1969; 1971) using the "choral" method previously described by Tarnoczy (1958) for measurements on groups of speakers. All these methods are being used for speech analysis in different applications which can be broadly classified as diagnostic, or for assessment of the effects of treatment.

DIAGNOSTIC APPLICATIONS

One of the first medical uses of speech analysis was in psychiatry when Zwirner (1930) analysed the speech of a group of depressives to study their apparent monotony. Luchsinger and Brunner (1950) investigated the monotonous speech of epileptics and since then many other psychiatrists including Ostwald (1965) have used analysis of speech to monitor emotional states. Simonov (1969) claims that analysis of voice pattern is a more sensitive test of the effect of stress than psychiatric evaluation and revealed that Russian cosmonauts are checked for emotional stability by analysis of their speech. Furthermore Rousey (1970) has proposed speech analysis for use in community mental health screening centres.

According to Friedman *et al.* (1969), subjects who show a behaviour pattern associated with a high prevalence and incidence rate of coronary heart disease can be identified by analysis of their speech during "hortatory" reading. Subjects with this particular behaviour pattern are found to have explosive vocal intonations which can be measured from recordings of their speech.

Lind (1971) finds that spectrographic analysis of the cry of the newborn child yields diagnostic information in conditions including chromosomal anomalies (cat-cry disease, Down's syndrome, etc.), cerebral damage from birth trauma (anoxia and haemorrhage), hyperbilirubinuria with cerebral involvement, newborn hypoglycaemia and meningitis.

As a diagnostic aid to the laryngologist, using modern electroacoustical techniques, it is possible to measure the small acoustical changes which result from polyps and inflammation on or around the vocal cords, carcinoma in the larynx and on the vocal cords. Bowler (1964) reported that hoarse voices are associated with "breaks" in the fundamental frequencies and variations in the periodicities of the acoustic waveform. This discovery has been followed up by von Leden and Koike (1970) who measured some 30 consecutive periods of the fundamental in a sustained vowel sound written out by an ultra-violet recorder; a PDP 8 digital computer was then used to extract the pitch perturbations by auto-correlation techniques. Four grades of perturbation were distinguished in different patients with degrees of laryngeal pathology of increasing severity. Iwata and von Leden (1970) have used contour spectrograms in a parallel study of hoarse voices. They found that fluctuation of the fundamental frequency was more easily detected in this form of presentation than with the bar spectrograms previously employed.

In an application of speech analysis to screening populations for laryngeal disorders, Smith and Lieberman (1969) reported that a small portable computer-type unit was being developed in the United States to measure a subject's pitch information, compare it with stored patterns of known characteristics, and print out a diagnosis. This followed trials involving tedious measurement of individual periods of the waveform and punching the data on to IBM cards for processing in an IBM 7090 computer to obtain the distribution of variations in pitch periods. Similar studies are being conducted at the Institute of Laryngology and Otology with the help of the Medical Research Council's Computer Services Centre and the Department of Electrical Engineering at Imperial College. An IBM 1800 computer is being used for direct analogue to digital conversion of sustained vowel sounds of normals and of patients with known laryngeal pathology for detailed analysis on an IBM 360/65 computer at University College. The scope of indirect laryngoscopy also has been considerably extended in recent years by application of electro-acoustic methods to illuminate the movements of the vocal cords stroboscopically and so enable all phases of their vibration to be examined during phonation. A development has been the introduction of the voice-controlled light source into an operating microscope recently described by McKelvie *et al.* (1970).

Another field to which speech spectrograms, or voiceprints, have been applied by Kersta (1962) is that of voice identification for law enforcement and other purposes. Speech spectrograms were admitted as evidence in a Court of Law in the United States in 1966. They were employed in 1967 to substantiate the claim of the Israeli Government that it had intercepted a radio-telephone conversation between President Nasser and King Hussein in which the Egyptian President claimed that U.S.A.F. and R.A.F. aircraft assisted the Israeli Forces. Since then speech scientists and acousticians in many countries have been requested to attempt the identification of recorded telephone threats, etc., with a recording of a suspect's voice. There are many difficulties in such a procedure, however, and a review of the reliability of the method was recently published which had been commissioned by a committee of the Acoustical Society of America (Bolt *et al.*, 1970).

ASSESSMENT OF THE EFFECTIVENESS OF TREATMENT

Considerable research has been conducted into the more severely disordered forms of speech which occur in the oesophageal speech of subjects after surgical removal of the larynx (Tato *et al.*, 1954; Van Den Berg *et al.*, 1958; Kytta, 1964; Hoops and Noll, 1969). Similarly, the acoustic characteristics of the speech of the deaf and partially-hearing has been studied by Penn (1955), Lindner (1956) and Hood and Dixon (1969). Lehiste (1965) has reviewed the properties of other forms of dysarthric speech. With existing methods of speech analysis, the means are already available to enable objective measurements in acoustical terms to be made of improvements resulting from treatment. Increasing use is being made of computers in these investigations and a study just started in New York is to provide basic information for developing better aids in teaching the deaf to speak. Computer correlations will be obtained between perceptual evaluation of deaf children's speech and physical quantification of the speech sounds by computer. The New York study, in common with the screening for laryngeal disorders research already mentioned, is supported by the U.S. Department of Health, Education and Welfare, and involves a total investment of $400,000 in the development of these two uses of speech analysis.

Apart from the obvious application of speech analysis techniques for objective estimation of improvement or deterioration as a result of treatment in psychiatric disease, other possible fields of interest are in the treatment of Parkinson's disease, in monitoring the virilizing side-effects in women of anabolic steroids and of dysfunction of the endocrine glands. The same electro-acoustic techniques can be employed with advantage to investigate all other body sounds. For example, in dentistry, Watt (1970) studied the sounds of occlusion of the teeth to relate the types of tooth contact which produced them, and he hopes by this means to predict occlusal disturbances before they can be detected visually. However, the sounds most frequently investigated diagnostically in medical practice are those produced within the heart and the lungs and, in the past, they have been assessed subjectively often by means of stethoscopes of variable and low-quality acoustic characteristics (Hollins, 1971). Already physicians are recording, with contact microphones, the sounds of respiration in some cases with a view to using acoustic means to locate the exact source of the component sounds and, in others, to compare the effects of different treatments. Heart sounds and murmurs are being treated in the same way. In Vienna, cardiologists are using a Real Time Analyzer to monitor the sound spectrum of heart sounds of patients with artificial mitral or aortic valves. It is possible in this way to detect wear in the artificial valves at an early stage (Brüel and Kjaer, 1971). Here it can be said that in one respect the wheel has turned a full circle, for it was from a study of a means of improving the electro-acoustic examination of heart murmurs 40 years ago that Dr T. S. Littler (whose name has been commemorated in their Society Awards at this Conference) turned his attention to Audiology.

ACKNOWLEDGEMENTS

The support of a grant G.969/406/C from the Medical Research Council is gratefully acknowledged. Thanks are also due to Mr C. J. North who provided the speech spectrogram of Fig. 1 and to the Voiceprint Laboratories of Somerville, New Jersey, U.S.A. for Fig. 2.

REFERENCES

Bolt, R. H., Cooper, F. S., David, E. E., Denes, P. B., Pickett, J. M. and Stevens, K. N. (1970). *J. acoust. Soc. Am.*, **47**, 597.

Bordone-Sacerdote, C. and Sacerdote, G. G. (1969). *Acustica*, **21**, 191.

Bordone-Sacerdote, C. and Sacerdote, G. G. (1971). *J. Aud. Technique*, **7**, 1.

Bowler, N. W. (1964). *Speech Monog.*, **31**, 128.

Brüel and Kjaer (1971). "Application Notes on Real Time Analyzer Type 3347". Naerum, Denmark.

Fourcin, A. J. and Abberton, E. (1971). *Med. Biol. Illustr.*, **21**, 172.

Friedman, M., Brown, A. E. and Rosenman, R. H. (1969). *J. Am. med. Assoc.*, **208**, 828.

Hollins, P. J. (1971). *Brit. J. hosp. Med.*, **5**, 509.

Hood, R. B. and Dixon, R. F. (1969). *J. Commun. Dis.*, **2**, 20.

Hoops, H. R. and Noll, J. D. (1969). *J. Commun. Dis.*, **2**, 1.

Iwata, S. and Leden, von H. (1970). *Arch. Otolaryng.*, **91**, 346.

Kersta, L. G. (1962). *Nature*, **196**, 1253.

Kytta, J. (1964). *Acta Otolaryng.* Suppl., 195.

Leden, H. von and Koike, Y. (1970). *Arch. Otolaryng.*, **91**, 3.

Lehiste, I. (1965). *Bibliotheca Phonetica* No. 2.

Lind, J. (1971). *Proc. R. Soc. Med.*, **64**, 468.

Lindner, G. (1956). *Arch. Ohr. Nas. Kehlkopfh.*, **169**, 557.

Luchsinger, R. and Brunner, R. (1950). *Folia Phoniat.*, **2**, 79.

McKelvie, P. and North, C. J. (1970). *Lancet*, ii, 503.

Ostwald, P. F. (1965). *Scient. Am.*, p. 82, March.

Penn, J. P. (1955). *Acta Otolaryng.* Suppl., 124.

Rousey, C. (1960). Reported in, *Med. News Tribune*, **2**, 1.

Simonov, P. V. (1969). Reported in, *Wld Med.*, **4**, No. 24.

Smith, W. R. and Lieberman, P. (1969). *Computers Biomed. Res.*, **2**, 291.

Tarnóczy, T. (1958). *Acustica*, **8**, 352.

Tato, J. M., Mariana, N., Picolli, de E., and Mirasov, P. (1954). *Acta Otolaryng.* **44**, 431.

Van Den Berg, J. Moolenaar-Bijl, A. and Damste, P. H. (1958). *Folia Phoniat.*, **10**, 65.

Watt, D. M. (1970). *Proc. R. Soc. Med.*, **63**, 793.

Zwirner, E. (1930). *J. Psychiatrie. Neurol.*, **41**, 43.

A Clinical Evaluation of the SAL Test

G. W. GLOVER and I. A. STEWART

Department of Otolaryngology, University of Dundee,
Dundee, Scotland

The Sensori-neural Acuity Level Test (or SAL Test) was introduced by Jerger and Tillman (1960). It was proposed as a simplification of the somewhat cumbersome technique described by Rainville (1955). The test is claimed to overcome certain problems in conventional bone conduction audiometry, particularly that of masking the non-test ear.

The Sensori-neural Acuity Level is assessed by determining the degree to which an air-conducted pure-tone signal is masked by a thermal noise delivered directly to the cochlea via bone conduction. The BC vibrator is placed in the centre of the forehead (Fig. 1).

Figure 2 shows the following points in the normal right ear.

1. AC threshold, marked conventionally.
2. Forehead masking level at each frequency.
3. The threshold shift produced by this masking level shown graphically by the letter "S" and numerically at the foot for each frequency.

The threshold shift produced is related to the degree of sensori-neural hearing loss.

Taking single frequency examples (Fig. 3), it is seen in the normal that a 100 dB forehead masking level produces a shift of 40 dB; that is from 0–40.

In a conductive loss of 30 dB, the shift produced is also 40 dB; that is from 30–70.

In a sensori-neural loss of 30 dB, the shift produced is 10 dB; that is from 30–40.

This demonstrates the basis of the SAL test: the threshold shift produced in the subject is compared to the threshold shift in the normal.

Thus the shift produced in a conductive loss with an intact cochlea is

211

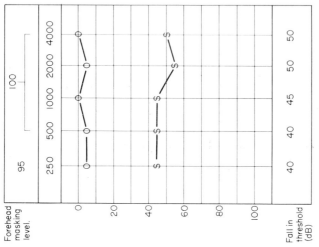

Fig. 2.

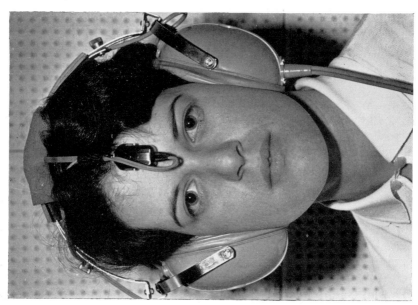

Fig. 1. This demonstrates: standard BC vibrator on the forehead; foam rubber insulation between vibrator and head set; the use of Sharpe ear-phones.

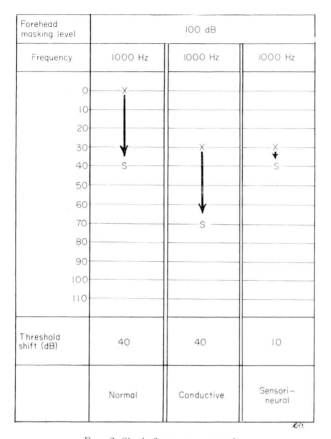

Forehead masking level	100 dB		
Frequency	1000 Hz	1000 Hz	1000 Hz
Threshold shift (dB)	40	40	10
	Normal	Conductive	Sensori-neural

F IG . 3. Single frequency examples.

identical to the shift in the normal, whereas in a sensori-neural loss the shift will be less.

It is obvious from this that the test must first be standardized in normals.

Problems arising from the original technique have been discussed by Tillman (1962). He demonstrated that by using Sharpe ear-phones, the errors produced by occlusion in the lower frequencies could be minimized. He also advocated the use of narrow band masking. His suggestions were adopted for this clinical trial.

The SAL test was attractive to us in that it apparently overcame the difficulties of masking the non-test ear, always a problem in conventional BC audiometry. The test also seemed simple and rapid to perform, thus being suited to the needs of a busy service clinic. No special equipment was necsssary.

Our first objective was to produce a normal series of threshold shifts for purposes of comparison to abnormals. It is interesting to note that no previous author has to our knowledge published detailed figures, "mean threshold shifts" always being quoted.

The histograms shown in Figs 4–8 depict the threshold shifts at each frequency obtained in 20 normals, i.e. 40 ears, using high level masking. The mean threshold shifts are marked beneath each, for example, at 1,000 Hz the shift is 57·5 dB. The wide scatter of results

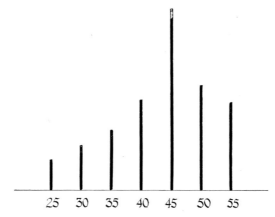

Fig. 4. 250 Hz. Mean threshold shift: 42·85 dB. Range: 25–55 dB.

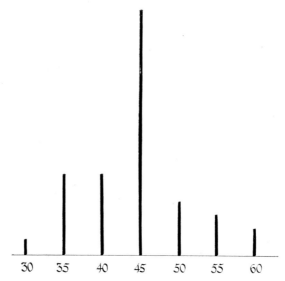

Fig. 5. 500 Hz. Mean threshold shift: 43·86 dB. Range 30–60 dB.

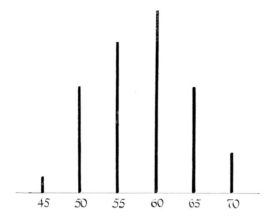

Fɪɢ. 6. 1 kHz. Mean threshold shift: 57·5 dB. Range: 45–70 dB.

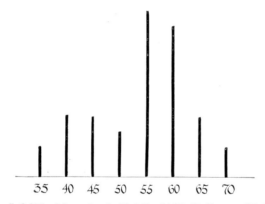

Fɪɢ. 7. 2 kHz. Mean threshold shift: 54·12 dB. Range: 35–70 dB.

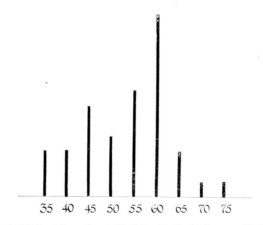

Fɪɢ. 8. 4 kHz. Mean threshold shift: 50·72 dB. Range: 35–75 dB.

obtained at all frequencies should be noted; thus at 250 Hz the range is from 25–55 dB and at 4,000 Hz from 35–75 dB.

By contrast there is close correlation between ears in any one individual as Fig. 9 shows. Thus out of 100 comparisons, only 3 per cent exceed 5 dB variation and none exceed 10 dB.

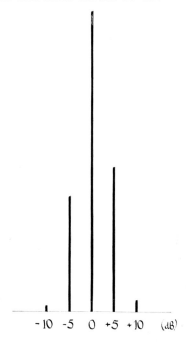

-10 -5   0   +5 +10   (dB)

Fɪɢ. 9. Variation between right and left ears in 20 normals.

Figure 10 compares the threshold shifts obtained in six normal individuals with a two-week interval between measurement. Therefore, results in one individual, although broadly comparable, are not absolutely reproducible. The reasons for such variations as do occur will be discussed.

Thus there is wide variation between individuals, some temporal variation, but close correlation between ears of any one individual on any one occasion.

The major question which arises is "Why this variation between individuals?"

Variations in transmission may result from the following factors.

1. Tension and position of BC head-band.
2. Variations in shape and size of head.
3. Thickness of subcutaneous tissues.

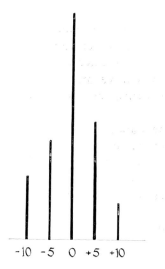

F IG. 10. Comparison of threshold shifts in six normals after a two-week interval.

4. Aeration of frontal sinuses.
5. Bone density.

The only one of these five factors open to technical error or variation is the application of the BC vibrator. We were careful to ensure good apposition of the vibrator to the forehead. We found that slight variations in position and pressure of the BC vibrator could result in a difference of up to 20 dB in any one individual. Care in application of the vibrator reduced these variations considerably, but this is obviously the cause of the temporal variations discovered. The anatomical factors are presumed to be the major cause of variation between individuals.

We would accordingly deduce that, at least in our hands, the SAL test as originally described is not acceptable, the reason being the wide variation in normals.

Our initial feeling of disappointment with these results was modified when we appreciated the highly significant correlation between ears in an individual. Although we did not consider that the test was acceptable as a routine method of measuring cochlear function, we considered that it could be validly modified to compare the two cochleas of an individual.

Using conventional techniques few problems arise in determining AC thresholds. The BC threshold of the better ear also rarely presents problems. Using the "modified SAL" technique which we will now describe, we have a test which is simple (compared to the Rainville test) and which is of some clinical value.

The technique is as follows:

An accurate AC level is determined using masking where appropriate. Using forehead masking at appropriate high levels the drop in AC at each frequency is determined for each ear in turn. The difference in threshold shifts is a relative measure of the difference in cochlear sensitivity. The sensori-neural level is then deduced from the BC curve of the better ear.

Figure 11 shows the standard form used for recording SAL results. The bottom left shows the conventional audiogram. Above, readings are depicted for the right and left ear, AC thresholds being depicted conventionally. The forehead masking level is recorded. The threshold shift produced by this is recorded graphically by the letter "S" and numerically below. In this oversimplified example, 100 dB of forehead masking is applied to ears which have respectively 20 dB and 40 dB sensori-neural loss. The threshold shift in the right ear is from 20–50 and that in the left ear from 40–50, i.e. the right ear is shifted 30 dB and the left ear 10 dB.

By subtraction (30–10), the sensori-neural difference is 20 dB.

The BC in the better ear is readily determinable, 20 dB; and the BC in the worse ear may be accordingly deduced—the sensori-neural difference being added to the BC threshold in the better ear, 20 + 20 = 40; and shown on the SAL predicted audiogram, bottom right. The conventional BC may then be compared to the SAL BC.

CLINICAL EXAMPLES

Case 1

This patient (Fig. 12) presented with recent right-sided deafness, tinnitus and vertigo. Initially his symptoms were thought to be Eustachian in origin as diagnostic myringotomy produced serious fluid. Treatment resulted in a normal drum but his symptoms persisted. Using the SAL technique there was no threshold shift in the right ear. The sensori-neural difference as calculated demonstrates that the loss must be greater than that measured conventionally. For example, at 500 Hz, the threshold shift in the left ear is 45 dB. The sensori-neural difference between the ears (45–0) is 45 dB. This is added to the BC threshold in the better ear; 15 + 45 is 60 dB. The modified SAL thus predicts a loss of greater than 60 dB. In other words, the SAL confirms the sensori-neural loss suggested by the tuning fork tests. The conventional audiogram is a misrepresentation, presumably due to inadequate masking or pallaesthesia.

To divert for a moment here, we would like to point out that BC

UNIVERSITY OF DUNDEE
DEPARTMENT OF OTOLARYNGOLOGY
S. A. L. ASSESSMENT RECORD

Name _TYPE EXAMPLE_ _____ Age _____ Sex _____ Unit No. _____

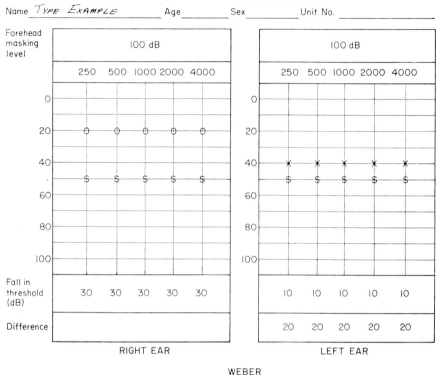

RIGHT EAR   LEFT EAR

WEBER

RINNE.

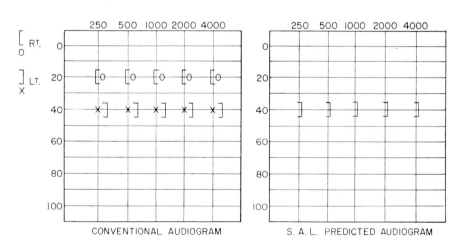

CONVENTIONAL AUDIOGRAM   S. A. L. PREDICTED AUDIOGRAM

Fɪɢ. 11. Modified SAL record form.

Name J. STIRLING   Age 37   Sex M.   Unit No. 89535

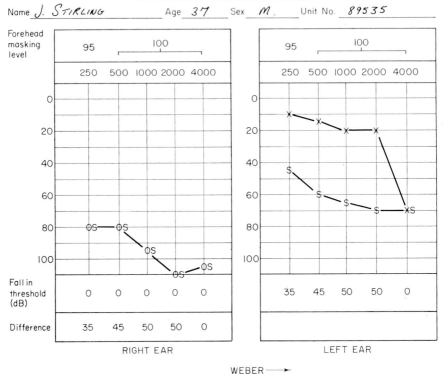

WEBER ⟶

False neg. RINNE. +

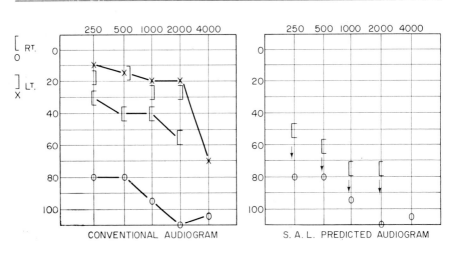

Fɪɢ. 12.

masking techniques overcome the problem of pallaesthesia, i.e. false responses mediated via the vibration sense, particularly in the low frequencies.

Case 2

This young woman (Fig. 13) has been deaf in her right ear since childhood. The tympanic membrane was normal. Her conventional audiogram is shown bottom left. Her SAL predicted audiogram is similar and thereby confirms a result which initially appeared dubious. It also demonstrates the BC responses are not Pallaesthesia.

Case 3

This patient (Fig. 14) presented with right-sided deafness dating from a mastoidectomy in infancy. His conventional audiogram suggested some sensori-neural loss, although he referred his Weber to the right. The clinical suspicion was of a dislocated incus. We were hesitant to re-explore the ear in the presence of a sensori-neural loss. The upper two audiograms show threshold shifts in the right and left ears. You will note only 70 dB of masking was used, as higher masking levels depressed the threshold beyond the limit of the audiometer.

Our SAL predicted audiogram demonstrates that cochlear impairment is minimal.

Case 4

This man (Fig. 15) presented with right-sided deafness, with recent rapid progression. The conventional audiogram and his history of sinus disease suggested a conductive component. The drum was thickened and poorly mobile. Inflation did not improve his symptoms.

The SAL technique demonstrates again that this is sensori-neural, the conventional audiogram presumably being fallacious.

Case 5

This (Fig. 16) is the audiogram of one of the authors (I.A.S.), who has a dead ear on the right. The curve shown on the left audiogram is a "shadow curve" obtained without masking the left ear. High level forehead masking completely masked the dead ear at all frequencies other than 500 Hz, the circled S.

This is of relevance to the problem of shadow curves with the SAL technique. Thus comparing left with right at 2,000 Hz, the inter-aural attenuation is 65 dB. The shift with forehead masking is 60 dB making a total of 125 dB, which is the effective isolation between the two ears.

By contrast at 500 Hz the inter-aural attenuation is 60 dB and the

UNIVERSITY OF DUNDEE
DEPARTMENT OF OTOLARYNGOLOGY
S. A. L. ASSESSMENT RECORD

Name J. HEALD   Age 23   Sex F   Unit No. 253559

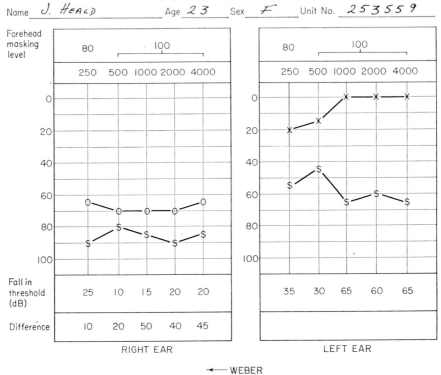

RIGHT EAR   LEFT EAR

◄── WEBER

Neg. RINNE. Pos.

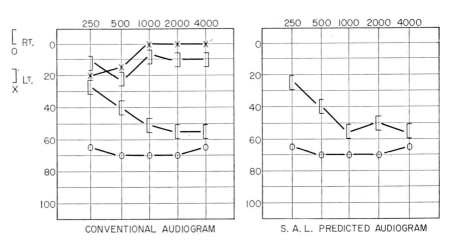

CONVENTIONAL AUDIOGRAM   S. A. L. PREDICTED AUDIOGRAM

FIG. 13.

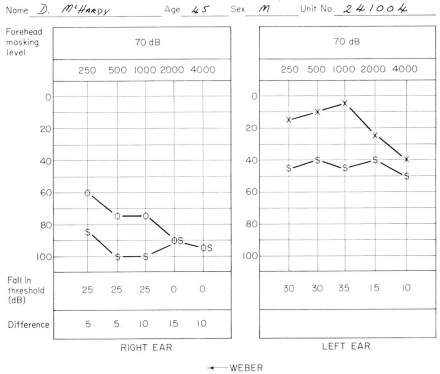

UNIVERSITY OF DUNDEE
DEPARTMENT OF OTOLARYNGOLOGY
S. A. L. ASSESSMENT RECORD

Name _D. McHARDY_   Age _45_   Sex _M_   Unit No. _241004_

Forehead masking level	70 dB					70 dB				
	250	500	1000	2000	4000	250	500	1000	2000	4000
Fall in threshold (dB)	25	25	25	0	0	30	30	35	15	10
Difference	5	5.	10	15	10					
	RIGHT EAR					LEFT EAR				

 WEBER

Neg. RINNE. Pos.

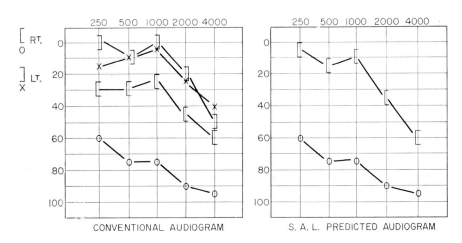

CONVENTIONAL AUDIOGRAM   S. A. L. PREDICTED AUDIOGRAM

FIG. 14.

Name W. CARR   Age 68   Sex M   Unit No. 27512

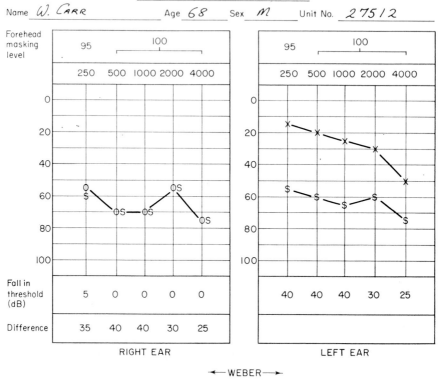

RIGHT EAR   LEFT EAR

←—WEBER—→
+ RINNE. +

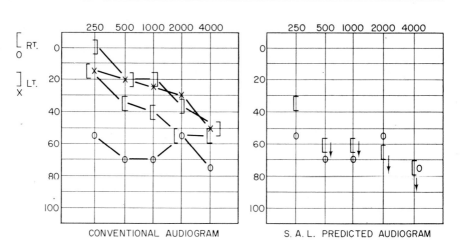

CONVENTIONAL AUDIOGRAM   S. A. L. PREDICTED AUDIOGRAM

FIG. 15.

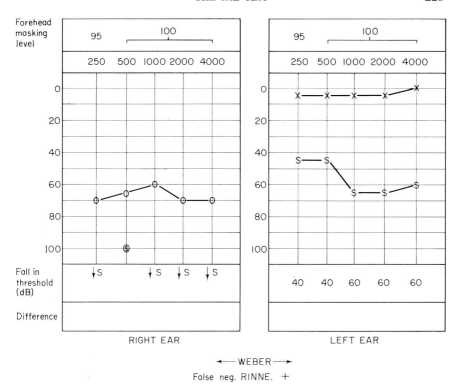

shift 40 dB, making a total of 100 dB. You will note that a shadow recording was obtained at this level (100 dB). To generalize from this, the effective isolation between ears is predictable in this way. With high forehead masking levels shadow curves are rarely a problem. A suspected shadow curve could be excluded by additional insert masking, but this would so complicate the test as to make it of less value.

CONCLUSION

In summary, these are the advantages and disadvantages of the "modified SAL".

Advantages
1. Overcomes the masking problem.
2. Eliminates pallaesthesia.
3. Eliminates standardization with normals.
4. Eliminates variables of the siting of BC vibrator.
5. Allows for shadow curves.
6. Does not require high degree of audiometric skill.

7. Quick.
8. Utilizes standard equipment.

Disadvantages

1. The problem of occlusion (this is largely eliminated by Sharpe ear-phones).
2. Maximum measurable sensori-neural loss limited by threshold shift in better ear.
3. Allowance for shadow curves complicates the test.
4. Use of high voltage across BC terminals causing overloading. This may affect calibration of the audiometer.

The SAL test as originally described was advocated as a convenient substitute for conventional BC audiometry. We cannot accept this. We would however feel justified in concluding that this modification of the SAL test may usefully complement the conventional audiogram and clinical findings, particularly in difficult cases.

ACKNOWLEDGEMENTS

We would like to thank Mr A. G. Gibb, Head of the Department of Otolaryngo-logy, University of Dundee, for his active encouragement. The "S" notation used for depicting threshold shift is the idea of Mr A. Blick. Alfred Peters provided the Sharpe ear-phones

REFERENCES

Jerger, J. F. and Tillman, T. (1960). *Archs. Otolar.*, **71**, 948.
Tillman, T. (1962). Tech. Doc. Rep. School of Aerospace Medicine, *T.D.R.*, 62–96.
Rainville, M. J. (1955). *J. franc. otolaryng.*, **4**, 851.

Computer Analysis of Audiological Aspects of Otosclerosis

A. G. GIBB and R. K. MAL
Department of Otolaryngology, University of Dundee,
Dundee, Scotland,

INTRODUCTION

Audiology can play a useful role in throwing light on certain of the problems facing the clinician. The accurate correlation of clinical findings, pathological changes and audiological data is an intriguing and at times rewarding exercise to the otologist.

The investigations outlined in this paper relate to specific audiological aspects of a wider survey on otosclerosis.

METHODS OF INVESTIGATION

In 1969, an investigation was commenced on a series of stapedectomy operations carried out by one of us (A.G.G.). This involved the analysis of 337 cases operated on over a period of approximately nine years. As so often happens the more deeply the problem was investigated the more involved it became, until it grew obvious that a computer study offered the most logical method of sifting the mass of diverse information already collected. Although the survey is now a continuing one, the initial analysis was carried out retrospectively, despite the drawbacks and limitations of such a procedure of which we were fully aware. The information on which the study was based was mainly obtained from the case records but a questionnaire was also circulated, to confirm and supplement certain aspects of the information already obtained. Data processing was carried out using an I.C.L. 1901A computer.

Computer analysis proved not only a convenient method of evaluating and comparing different stapedectomy techniques but was also of inestimable value in the complicated task of assessing the significance of the clinical data in relation to the evolving audiometric pattern.

In planning the survey four main aspects received special attention:

1. Pre-operative assessment of the otosclerotic individual.
2. Detailed recording of operation findings.
3. Analysis of post-operative complications.
4. Recording of audiometric data.

AUDIOMETRIC DATA

In each case pure tone audiometry was carried out pre-operatively: in the later years of the survey speech discrimination scores were also recorded. Post-operatively, pure tone audiometry was undertaken after one month and thereafter at intervals of three months, six months and annually for five years. Quite a proportion of cases have actually been followed up with audiometry as long as eight years after operation but annual assessments after the five years' mark are not always practical nor in fact very informative. It is hoped, however, that in a relatively static community such as exists in and around Dundee a high proportion of ten-year results may eventually be obtainable.

INVESTIGATIONS RELATED TO PRE-OPERATIVE ASSESSMENT

Vertigo

It is generally accepted that vertiginous attacks encountered in otosclerosis result from recurring disturbances of the labyrinth directly related to the otosclerotic process. Keeping this concept in mind it was decided to find out if the cochlea in such cases was especially sensitive to operative trauma.

In this series 54 (18 per cent) cases complained of intermittent vertigo pre-operatively: post-operative audiometric recordings of this selected group failed to show any increased incidence of sensori-neural hearing loss. Indeed the attainment of the predicted hearing gain at operation was in no way influenced by the presence of pre-operative vertigo. (Fig. 1).

Tinnitus

Tinnitus is such a common symptom in otosclerosis (59 per cent of cases in this series) that it is obviously in the surgeon's interest to know whether cases with pre-operative tinnitus can anticipate comparable hearing gains to those without tinnitus. The two groups were therefore analysed and compared and the findings are shown in Fig. 2. The results suggest that cases with tinnitus tend if anything to obtain slightly greater hearing improvement than non-tinnitus cases especially in the higher frequencies. Too much significance, however, should not be attached to this finding as the trend is slight and the series as yet is

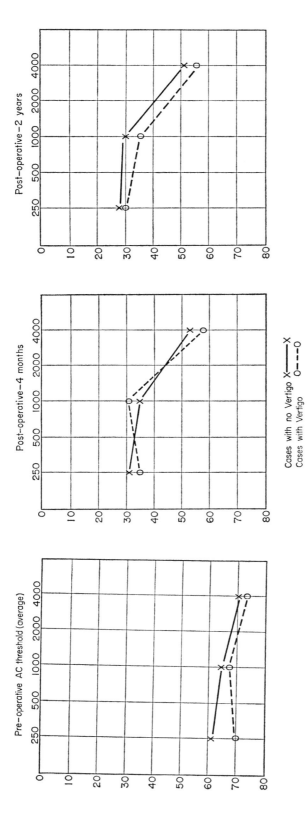

Fig. 1. Relationship of pre-operative vertigo to post-operative threshold shift.

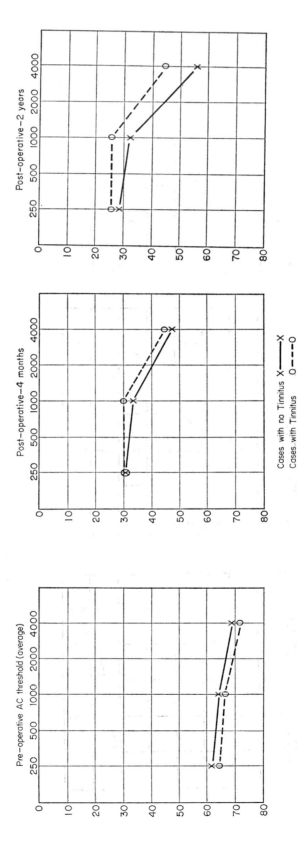

Fig. 2. Relationship of pre-operative tinnitus to post-operative threshold shift.

relatively small: later studies with a larger series of cases may prove of greater significance. A possible explanation for the present pattern might be that tinnitus obscures, and as a result depresses, the pre-operative audiometric threshold: if, after stapedectomy, the masking effect of the tinnitus is eliminated, the true audiometric threshold will be recorded, thus giving the impression of a greater hearing improvement than has actually occurred.

INVESTIGATIONS RELATED TO SURGICAL TECHNIQUE

There are many problems related to the stapedectomy operation but two only will be considered.

Blood in the Vestibule
Bleeding in the region of the oval window may complicate stapes surgery. If blood escapes into the vestibule the situation presents an urgent surgical problem requiring an immediate decision as to whether to aspirate the blood or allow it to remain in the vestibule. An analysis of the audiometric results was carried out in order to throw some light on this problem (Table I): the investigation findings suggested that the

TABLE I
The Influence on Hearing of Bleeding into the Vestibule

	Blood in Vestibule		
	Nil	Slight	Gross
No. of cases	83	167	19
AC Average*	39 dB	37 dB	42 dB

* Average of 5 frequencies, two years after operation.

presence of blood in the vestibule had very little effect on the ultimate hearing level: it would seem reasonable, therefore, to refrain from aspirating blood from the vestibule with all the attendant risks to inner ear structures. The above findings were not altogether unexpected since they were in accordance with the conclusions of Linthicum and Sheehy (1969) and the experimental work which they cite of Schuknecht.

Removal of Perilymph
Variable quantities of perilymph may be aspirated if suction is applied near the oval windows ranging from scarcely detectable amounts to the so-called "dry" vestibule. Opinions differ widely on the relative risks involved: a summation of the audiometric results in this survey showed

that as far as the post-operative hearing threshold was concerned the removal of perilymph had an almost negligible effect (Table II).

TABLE II

The Influence on Hearing of Removal of Perilymph

	Perilymph Loss		
	Nil	Slight	Gross
No. of Cases	98	48	121
AC Average*	36 dB	42 dB	38 dB

* Average over 5 frequencies: two years after operation.

INVESTIGATIONS RELATED TO POST-OPERATIVE ASSESSMENT

Exposure to Noise

In the East of Scotland region centred in Dundee, jute weaving with its related noise hazards is carried out almost exclusively by a female population. Since otosclerosis is also predominantly a disease of females an exceptional opportunity is afforded to study the hearing thresholds of stapedectomized subjects who subsequently return to a noisy environment.

In our investigations, 4 kHz was selected as the critical frequency in comparing cases working post-operatively in quiet surroundings with those in noisy environments. A comparison between these groups proved easy since, rather fortuitously, both showed a mean hearing loss of 56 dB four months after operation. At the end of five years the mean hearing threshold remained unaltered in either group (Table III).

TABLE III

Noise Exposure after Stapedectomy

	Pre-op		Post-operative			
			4 months	10 months	2 years	5 years
Cases without Noise exposure	70 dB (278)	O P E R A T I O N	56 dB (261)	48 dB (177)	51 dB (127)	56 dB (54)
Cases with Noise exposure	74 dB (39)		56 dB (36)	51 dB (26)	55 dB (21)	56 dB (16)

Average AC Thresholds at 4 kHz.
Figures in brackets refer to number of cases.

This result was somewhat surprising since we had expected the noise exposed group to show, at least, the usual threshold shift normally encountered in healthy ears. We can offer no ready explanation for this but it must be noted that glass down was prescribed post-operatively to reduce the noise hazard: we suspect, however, that in general it was used only in the early post-operative period.

Special problems might be expected since most operative techniques involve division of the stapedius tendon and the protective action of this muscle on the inner ear is consequently abolished. In actual fact, this procedure may have negligible sequelae as it is extremely doubtful if the stapedius has any significant protective role in *continuous* noise exposure since it is unlikely that the muscle can maintain a constant state of tonic contraction over long periods.

The role of stapedius in industrial noise was investigated by one of us (Gibb, 1964) when a small number of stapedectomy cases in which the stapedius had been divided, together with suitable controls, were exposed to industrial noise in a jute factory for a measured period of time. Both the stapedectomized and normal ears behaved identically, the induced temporary threshold shift being independent of the integrity of stapedius. If any stapedius function exists in industrial noise it is likely to be related only to peaks produced by impact noise.

In actual fact, in several cases in the present series it was possible either to lengthen and reconstruct the stapedius tendon (after Hough, personal communication) or retain it intact but with preservation of an ossicular attachment to the incus only (after Farrior, 1962). These techniques were utilized primarily to ensure an adequate vascular supply to the incus rather than to preserve a functioning stapedius. Even in the cases where the muscle was retained intact we do not believe that function was preserved as we were unable to demonstrate a sta-pedius reflex, by impedance audiometry, at least in the early post-operative period.

Changes in Bone Conduction Thresholds

With improving standards of education, more and more patients demand to know their chances of success, or failure, before undergoing any elective surgical procedure. This question is especially relevant in stapedectomy since the otologist is usually able to give an accurate prediction of the post-operative hearing improvement. In arriving at this assessment one of the most important factors—perhaps *the* most vital— is the state of the inner ear, since many otologists base their prognosis on the pattern of the air-bone gap, i.e. they reckon to bring the post-operative AC threshold up to the level of the pre-operative BC threshold, thus closing the gap. However if this method of assessment is employed, a latent problem exists since it has been shown by both

Carhart (1950) and McConnell (1950) that in cases of stapes fixation the bone conduction threshold, as determined by standard audiometric techniques, is not a true reflection of the cochlear reserve. The reasons for this remain the subject of controversy but are beyond the scope of this paper. Suffice it to state that Carhart estimated the BC threshold in stapes fixation to be depressed by the following amounts, 5 dB at 500 Hz, 10 dB at 1 kHz, 15 dB at 2 kHz and 5 dB at 4 kHz, the corresponding dip in the ordinary BC audiogram being commonly referred to as Carhart's notch. Thus to determine the true sensori-neural reserve in otosclerosis the BC curve must be "corrected" by adding the above amounts.

While not questioning the validity of the above figures we considered it necessary to find out if in practice the Carhart notch is abolished after a successful stapedectomy operation or if not, what bone conduction shift, if any, takes place. In this connection it was noteworthy that McConnell found that after fenestration operations Carhart's notch was only partially reversed. The effect of stapes mobilization on BC threshholds was the subject of disagreement for while Shambaugh (1959) reported cases in which the Carhart notch was completely reversed Rosen et al. (1959) failed to find improvement in BC thresholds after operation.

We therefore sought answers to the following questions in our efforts to arrive at as accurate a prognosis as possible in stapedectomy.

1. Should the pre-operative BC audiogram be corrected?
   If "yes"
2. What correction factor should be applied?
3. Should the same correction factor be applied to different patterns of otosclerotic deafness?

In this investigation only "successful" operation cases were included (i.e. cases with post-operative closure of the air-bone gap) as failures would merely have tended to distort the results.

A comparison between the pre-operative and post-operative BC thresholds clearly demonstrated that in the majority of cases BC thresholds were improved after operation especially at the 2 kHz and 4 kHz frequencies. Indeed the change in audiometric thresholds was so clear cut that it at once became obvious that a correction figure was not only justified but highly important in an accurate prediction of the outcome of stapedectomy. While it is appreciated that an average correction figure may not be appropriate for every case since the shift in BC responses is inconstant and varies from one patient to another, failure to make any correction adjustment would certainly result in borderline cases suitable for operation being excluded. However, the mean BC shift in this series was much less than Carhart's original estimate and the correction factor is correspondingly less and more in line with McConnell's figures for fenestration operations (Table IV).

TABLE IV

Estimated Correction Factor to Compensate for BC Shift in Stapes Fixation

	250 Hz	500 Hz	1 kHz	2 kHz	4 kHz
Carhart's estimate	0	5 dB	10 dB	15 dB	5 dB
Shift following fenestration (McConnell)	—	—	6·5 dB	8·5 dB	4·2 dB
Shift following stapedectomy*	0	2 dB	4 dB	8 dB	3 dB

* Average correction in present series based on multiple post-operative audiograms.

In determining whether the same correction factor should be applied to different patterns of otosclerosis it was argued that cases with a small air-bone gap might not necessarily have a completely fixed stapes and therefore the sensori-neural reserve would more closely approximate the curve of the standard BC audiogram. Cases with differing widths or air-bone gaps were therefore analysed in separate groups (under 30 dB, 31–40 dB and over 40 dB). All these groups were found to have similar BC shifts requiring the same correction curves. These findings supported the opinions of Graham (1953) and Carhart who contended that notching of the BC audiogram occurs at an early stage of the otosclerotic process before the stapes is completely fixed and therefore before the degree of deafness is likely to merit stapedectomy.

SUMMARY

A computer analysis of 337 cases of otosclerosis undergoing stapedectomy was carried out with the following results.

1. Pre-operative vertigo was not associated with an increased incidence of post-operative sensori-neural hearing loss.
2. Cases with pre-operative tinnitus had post-operative hearing gains slightly greater than average.
3. The operative complications of blood entering the vestibule and excessive removal of perilymph had no significant effect on the ultimate hearing result.
4. Patients working in noisy environments after operation showed no evidence of hearing regression at the 4 kHz frequency after five years. The reason for this finding was unexplained.

5. The existence of Carhart's notch was confirmed: post-operative BC shift was less than in Carhart's original estimate and the correction factor employed in predicting post-operative hearing improvement was correspondingly less: the same correction factor is applicable to different patterns of otosclerotic deafness irrespective of the width of the air-bone gap.

ACKNOWLEDGEMENTS

We acknowledge the assistance of the Eastern Regional Hospital Board (Scotland) in providing facilities and personnel for data processing.

REFERENCES

Carhart, R. (1950). Clinical application of bone conduction audiometry. *Arch. Otolaryng.*, **51**, 798.

Farrior, J. B. (1962). Stapedectomy and tympanoplasty. *Arch. Otolaryng.*, **76**, 140.

Gibb, A. G. (1964). Scottish Otolaryngological Society proceedings. *J. Laryng.*, **78**, 561.

Graham, A. B. (1953). An audiological and otological investigation of normal hearing individuals with a family history of clinical otosclerosis. Northwestern Univ. Ph.D. Thesis, Chicago.

Linthicum, F. H. and Sheehy, J. L. (1969). Blood in the vestibule at stapedectomy. *Ann. Otol. Rhinol. Laryngol.*, **78**, 425.

McConnell, F. E. (1950). Influence of fenestration surgery on bone conduction acuity. Northwestern University Ph.D. thesis, Chicago.

Rosen, S., Bergman, M. and Grossman, I. (1959). Bone conduction thresholds in stapes surgery. *Arch. Otolaryng.*, **70**, 365.

Shambaugh, G. E. (1959). "Surgery of the Ear", p. 344. W. B. Saunders Co., Philadelphia.

Neuro-Otolaryngology in West Africa

R. HINCHCLIFFE

*Institute of Laryngology and Otology, University of London,
London, England*

INTRODUCTION

West Africa is a well defined part of Africa. Desert separates it from
North Africa and the Cameroon, Bamenda and Adamawa mountains
keep it apart from the very different lowlands of West Central Africa.
Its coasts border on the Atlantic and they are more southern than
western. Historically, the empires of Ghana, Mali and Songhai span
the period from about the tenth to the fifteenth century. European
penetration was beginning in the middle of the nineteenth century and
if any one date were to mark its beginning it would be 1861 when
King Docemo ceded Lagos to the British. This year also marked the
beginnings of neuro-otolaryngology in Europe since it was then that
Ménière published his paper on the disorder which now bears his
name. Politically, West Africa was transformed from almost complete
colonialism in early 1957 to all but entire freedom a decade ago. Eco-
nomically, as Church (1967) points out, it is a major world producer and
seller of palm kernels and oil, cocoa, diamonds and manganese. The
Akosombo Dam of the Volta River Project in Ghana and the Kainji
Dam of Nigeria are associated with large hydro-electric power projects
which should transform West Africa. Medically, West Africa has now
emerged from the time when it was known as the "white man's grave",
but it still presents health problems associated with diseases which are
either unknown in Europe or occur on a different scale, and whose
nature now is only just beginning to be understood. Neuro-otolaryngology in particular presents many challenging problems.

This survey of neuro-otolaryngology in West Africa was prompted
by a Wellcome Trust-sponsored study visit to Ghana and Nigeria in
1970 at a time which coincided with the II Pan-African Conference of
Neurological Sciences, which enabled one to discuss general and
specific problems in this field.

237

HEARING AND SPEECH

One of the greatest problems is that of communication which is due to the large number of languages in the area. As Greenberg (1963) points out, the area contains languages from at least two totally unrelated language stocks, and a recent estimate by Ladefoged (1968) puts the total number of languages at well over 500. The multiplicity of languages has, however, provided useful material for study by linguists phoneticians and physicians. Ladefoged has made fundamental contributions to the subject of the phonetics of West African languages. Moreover, by investigating phenomena not present in European languages, the study was a contribution to phonetics in general and the methodology which he developed is applicable to research in phonetics in general.

The existence of a multiplicity of languages also implies that many of the people will be polyglots. Dada and his associates (1969) have made use of this in studying the effect of cerebrovascular accidents in such people to study the dissolution and recovery of language function. They have confirmed the previous finding of Pitres (1895) on Europeans that the polyglot who becomes aphasic and then recovers usually begins to understand and speak the language most familiar to him and in which he was most fluent at the onset of the aphasia, and not necessarily the language which he first learned.

Two recent hearing surveys (Reynaud et al., 1969; Hinchcliffe, et al., 1971) have left unresolved the question of whether or not the basic normal hearing levels of the African are better than those of his European counterpart. In both studies, a high prevalence of endemic disease was found and one wonders to what extent this has influenced the average hearing levels which were determined. One also wonders to what extent one was dealing with a survivor population as regards the older people, since Reynaud and his associates pointed out that the expectation of life in Senegal was 37 years. Nevertheless, a study of Simonetta (1968) of the Podokwo, who live on the eastern borders of this region, indicated that these people could hear sounds with frequencies as high as 24 kHz.

PATTERNS OF DISEASE

Trauma

Auditory and vestibular disorders arising from trauma are not uncommon. In clinics in the region where the author was able to observe patients, hearing losses due to direct trauma to the ear producing ruptured tympanic membranes were seen. In contrast to the condition in

Europe and North America, where occupational neuro-otological disorders are almost exclusively concerned with noise-induced hearing loss, auditory and vestibular disorders due to mechanical trauma are more conspicuous in this region. As Odeku and Richard (1970) pointed out, occupational trauma is a risk for two particular groups of individuals, i.e. palm tree tappers and load carriers. Tree falls by tappers can produce both traumatic hearing losses and vertigo and falls by load carriers can produce neck injuries which give rise to vertigo.

With the increase in industrialization associated particularly with the hydro-electric power projects, the relative prevalence of noise-induced hearing losses can be expected to rise.

Toxic Disorders

An endemic oto-neuro-ophthalmological syndrome, termed *Nigerian Nutritional Ataxia Neuropathy*, has been described in south-western Nigeria by Money (1958) and by Osuntokun (1968). In its fully developed extent, the syndrome comprises a myelopathy with predominant involvement of the posterior columns of the spinal cord, bilateral sensorineural hearing loss, optic atrophy and a symmetrical peripheral polyneuropathy. The condition is more prevalent in areas with a high cassava (*Manioc utilissima*) consumption (Osuntokun *et al.*, 1969), and is associated with high plasma thiocyanate levels (Monekosso and Wilson, 1966) and high blood free cyanide levels (Osuntokun *et al.*, 1970). Cassava contains high concentrations of a cyanogenetic glycoside, linamarin. The presumption is therefore that the disorder is due primarily to chronic cyanide intoxication, consequent on high cassava consumption. Experimental studies by Osuntokun and Williams (1970) have shown that rats fed on cassava preparations become ataxic and have higher plasma thiocyanate levels than control rats. Moreover, segmental demyelination was seen in the sciatic nerves of rats fed on the preparation for eighteen months.

A variety of audiometric patterns are observed in the syndrome and the topodiagnostic tests indicate the occurrence of both receptor organ and neuronal lesions (Hinchcliffe *et al.*, 1971). Evidence for auditory fatigue appeared to be associated with untreated cases of the condition.

As Osuntokun (1969) points out, it would be unrealistic to abandon cassava as a food product. There are several suggestions as to how relatively cyanide-free cassava meals might be prepared (de Paula and Rangel, 1946). The production of such palatable and acceptable derivatives with protein supplements (Oke, 1966) would, at the moment, appear to be the best means of preventing the disorder. At the moment, the production of cassava is increasing at the expense of other staple foods and more tobacco, which is locally produced, is being smoked. Smoking produces a greater cyanide exposure so that one can only expect an increase in both the prevalence and severity of this oto-neuro-ophthal-mological syndrome.

Collomb and his associates (1967) have reported a syndrome similar to the Nigerian neuromyelopathy in Senegal. In that country, the staple food is millet which contains a cyanogenetic glycoside termed dhurrin (Sinclair and Jelliffe, 1961).

Nwokolo and Ekpechi (1966) have shown that there is a high pre-valence of *goitre* in the Nsukka area of eastern Nigeria and that this is also associated with the consumption of unfermented cassava. The pre-valence reaches a peak in Ette where the prevalence of visible goitre is 325/1,000. Experimental studies on rats indicate that cassava contains a goitrogen and the results suggest that this acts like one of the thionamide group of anti-thyroid drugs, e.g. thiouracil (Ekpechi, 1967).

Outbreaks of what is known locally as *"Ilesha shakes"*, or what has been termed *"ancephalitis tremens"* by Wright and Morley (1958), occur in and around Ilesha in September and October each year. Ilesha is a rural town of about 75,000 people situated about 120 km north-east of Ibadan. The condition is characterized by a sudden onset of vertigo, which usually wakes the patient up in the middle of the night, and this is followed by vomiting and, when the patient stands up, violent shaking. This generalized tremor is the most dramatic feature of the syndrome. As Wright and Morley point out, the tremor is most marked by any attempt at movement but is decreased on lying down and dis-appears during sleep. The tremors might be followed by aphasia and even unconsciousness. Nevertheless, the course is in general benign, re-covery being the rule. A few patients have died through the oral admini-stration of local medicine which has been aspirated. As well as the general body tremor, the tongue often shows a tremor and the eyes show conjugate and horizontal oscillations, the description of which conforms more to a pendular nystagmus than a vestibular nystagmus. One or two cases are said to have had a hearing loss. Some of the patients have difficulty urinating and urinary retention is said to occur in about 5 per cent of affected individuals. There are no other abnormal neurological signs. In general the patients are not pyrexial, the calcium level in the blood is normal and the cerebro-spinal fluid shows no abnormality. The investigation of the urine of two of Wright and Morley's patients for alkaloids was negative. The yearly epidemics are spread over a period of about six weeks and arise in two distinct waves, which might suggest an infective aetiology. Apart from a similar syndrome which is said to occur in Haiti, the disease description, particularly as regards the generalized tremor and the influence of relaxation and sleep, bears some distinct resemblances to Kuru (Zigas and Gajdusek, 1957), the "trembling disease" which infects the Fore tribe of New Guinea and which has now been demonstrated to be due to a "slow" virus. However, Kuru is a progressive disorder, usually proceeding to a fatal outcome within about nine months and is characterized by widespread degeneration of the cerebellum and extrapyramidal system. Owing to the benign nature of the condition, there are no necropsy descriptions for Ilesha shakes. Moreover, serological examinations have persistently failed to indicate a virus aetiology. A virus has been isolated on one occasion only and it has not been possible to establish a connection between this virus and the disorder. All the affected individuals gave a history of eating pounded new yams (this is the season for new yams) so that a toxic aetiology is now thought to be a possibility. Although Hill (1952) has stated that there is a high concentration of cyanogenetic glycosides in some species of yams, analysis of *Dioscorea rotundata* in West Africa has failed to demonstrate any cyanide constituents. In any case, the clinical picture is not that of cyanide poisoning, so that one should look for other toxic chemicals. In particular, one should look to the metabolism of monoamines in affected subjects.

This treatment of affected individuals is admission to hospital and control of the shaking with chlorpromazine injections. The tremors abate within five days.

Deficiency Disorders

As Borgstrom (1969) has pointed out, mankind has already overextended itself and the developing world is on the brink of history's largest ever famine. Nigeria is no exception. Sales of Nigerian groundnuts on the world's markets deprive the country of an amount of protein which is about half of what is needed to fill the present protein gap. Protein deficiency is probably a factor in the aetiology of the ataxic neuromyelopathic syndromes. Collomb and his associates (1967) noted protein malnutrition in their patients. In discussing Nigerian Ataxic Neuropathy, Monekosso and Wilson (1966) pointed out that the detoxification of cyanide to thiocyanate must inevitably cause a further demand for sulphur-containing amino acids, providing an additional nutritional stress in people whose intake of protein is already low.

In Nigeria, Caddell (1966) has reported a *magnesium deficiency syndrome* which is characterized by spontaneous nystagmus, sensory ataxia and tremors or convulsions. The condition occurs in malnourished young children who have had severe prolonged gastro-enteritis and who have received a diet composed of corn starch and cassava. The condition is aggravated by vitamin B-enriched protein-milk therapy. The magnesium deficiency is established by biochemical analysis of skeletal muscle and of plasma. The symptoms are reversed by adding magnesium to food. Cassava and corn starch contain very little magnesium. It should be noted that magnesium plays an essential role in the biosynthesis and activation of thiamine pyrophosphate (Brown, 1960).

Genetically-determined Disorders

Otosclerosis is rarely encountered in the African but profound congenital sensorineural hearing loss is at least as common as it is in the United Kingdom and there are foci, as at Adamarobe in Ghana where the prevalence is extremely high (David *et al.*, 1971).

Heredo-degenerative disorders of the nervous system occur in the African (Collomb *et al.*, 1968) and geographical clusterings which occur in Senegal are due to consanguinity (Dumas *et al.*, 1968). In addition, Collomb and his associates (1967) have reported that there are ethnic differences in the patterns of the ataxic neuromvelopathic syndrome which is seen in Senegal. These differences may, of course, represent not the influence of genetic factors, but the influence of different geogens. Nevertheless, Behrman (1962) argues that there are genetic factors in the aetiology of tropical amblyopia, which, it might be contended, is a forme fruste of the tropical ataxic oto-neuro-ophthalmological syndrome.

Infective Disorders

Since otosclerosis and secretory otitis media are rarely encountered in the African, middle-ear infections remain the almost exclusive cause of conductive type hearing losses. Chronic middle-ear infections tend to present at a more advanced stage than they do in Britain, although the epitympanic type of cholesteatoma is less common. Tuberculosis is not an uncommon cause of middle ear disease in Nigeria but it is not characterized by the multiple tympanic membrane perforations which are described in textbooks of otology. The diagnosis in these cases is made by noting the watery discharge, the pale granulations and the radiological appearance of the lungs.

Sudden hearing loss is common in children but uncommon in adults in the region. The onset of the loss is usually associated with convulsions and a pyrexia. A viral aetiology is suspect.

In the more northerly areas of the region, meningitis is endemic, with periodic epidemics of both meningococcal and pneumococcal types. These infections are responsible for cases of profound sensori-neural hearing loss. In addition, in Nigeria, a *rapidly progressing sensori-neural hearing loss*, extending to sub-total loss over months or a year, afflicts teenagers and young adults in Nigeria. The aetiology of this has not yet been determined. Hearing losses due to either late congenital or acquired syphilis are rarely seen in the south of Nigeria. This is un-doubtedly due, at least in part, to the protective action of yaws. As in other parts of the world, an inverse prevalence of yaws and syphilis exist between northern and southern Nigeria (Findlay, 1946).

Lassa Fever is a particularly lethal (mortality estimated to be some-where between 50 and 80 per cent) infection which is named after the Nigerian village where it was first reported about two years ago. (Buckley and Casals, 1970; Frame *et al.*, 1970; Speir *et al.*, 1970; Troup *et al.*, 1970.) Lassa (10° 16′ N 13° 18′ E) is a village of about 1,000 people on the eastern border of northern Nigeria and lying in the Yedseram River Valley in the northern foothills of the Cameroons Highlands. Yale University Arborvirus Research Unit have shown that the infection is due to a virus which is similar in morphology, and re-lated antigenically, to the virus of lymphocytic choriomeningitis, as well as to those of Argentinian haemorrhagic fever (Junin) and Bolivian haemorrhagic fever (Machupo). The virus produces a fever as high as 107°, mouth ulcers, a skin rash with petechiae, pneumonia, infection of the heart leading to cardiac failure, kidney damage and severe muscle aches. One woman who recovered said "my eyes kept jerking from side to side and I could not watch television so I listened to my favourite hymns on the radio" (Article, *Daily Telegraph*, 1970). An examination of this patient showed her to have an ill-defined ocular jerky movement which could be classified neither as a pendular nor a vestibular nystag-mus. One woman who two years previously in Nigeria had suffered a similar illness which produced permanent bilateral deafness has been shown to have a high titre of antibodies for the virus. A hearing loss is now considered to be associated with a high proportion of cases of Lassa fever.

Neoplasms

Of 134 Nigerians who had intracranial tumours, one had a stato-acoustic nerve tumour. This tumour was bilateral and was associated with von Recklinghausen's disease (Odeku *et al.*, 1970). Girard and his associates (1970) reported that three out of 120 intracranial tumours observed in Senegal were stato-acoustic schwannomas. This data would therefore suggest that the prevalence of stato-acoustic tumours is no different from that in Europe and North America.

Other Disorders

Ménière's disorder is rare in West Africa (Osuntokun and Adeuja, 1970).

It is probable that Nigerian and other nutritional ataxic neuromyelo-pathies are not uncommon causes for recurrent vertigo in this region.

R

Although Williams and his associates (1969) have shown that the severity and extent of cerebral atherosclerosis in Nigerians is much less than it is in Euro-Americans and Afro-Americans, *degenerative vascular disease* may be a factor in the genesis of auditory and vestibular disorders in the elderly. For example, in Ghana I saw a 69-year-old female who had had an acute vestibular failure two weeks prior to my seeing her. Examination showed her to have a first degree spontaneous vestibular nystagmus to the right and a left canal paresis on the caloric test. The hearing was normal and there were no other neurological deficits.

Cases of combined *non-organic deafness and mutism* were observed in soldiers fighting in the Civil War in Nigeria. These patients responded to suggestion associated with the use of barbiturates intravenously.

Aural pain is a not uncommon symptom. At one otolaryngological clinic in Ghana where I was privileged to observe, five of the twenty-four outpatients seen in one session complained of aural pain. One of these was due to referred pain from a dental abscess, another was due to traumatic rupture of the eardrum, the third was due to an infected pre-auricular sinus, the fourth was due to keratosis obturans and the fifth to a seed impacted in the external meatus.

Tinnitus, with or without an associated hearing loss, presents a problem to the otologist in West Africa, just as much as it does to his colleagues in Europe. However, the difficulty is compounded in Nigeria by the Yoruba usually referring to the symptom as one of aural pain. Thus any patient complaining of aural pain in Nigeria must be asked "Does the pain make a noise or does it hurt?"

Facial nerve disorders, including Bell's palsy, are not uncommon. At the II Pan-African Congress of Neurological Sciences, Edoo (1970) reported a case of *epilepsia partialis continua* involving the left face. The electro-encephalograms in this case showed repeated spike discharges originating from the right frontal area, accompanied synchronously by artifacts of muscle spasm being picked up by the left scalp electrodes.

DIAGNOSTIC, THERAPEUTIC AND HABILITATIVE SERVICES

There is no doubt that personnel and facilities are inadequate for West Africa's needs. For example, in Nigeria, where the population is about the same size as that of the United Kingdom, there are only five otologists, a smaller number of neurologists and no audiologists in the country. Thus each specialist is responsible for at least twelve million people. With four otologists (two in Accra, one in Kumasi and one in

Tamale), Ghana fares somewhat better since her population is only about nine million. However, Ghana and Nigeria together have no more than six audiometers, half of which are probably unserviceable and the remainder have not been calibrated because of the absence of suitable facilities. Moreover, Nigeria does not yet possess any suitably acoustically-treated rooms for hearing tests. In Ibadan, however, there are facilities for elliptical tomography of the temporal bone (Lagundoye, 1971).

As Fiaxe (Commonwealth Society for the Deaf Report, 1968) and Ormerod (1961) point out, the first attempt to educate the deaf in Ghana was made in September 1957 when the Reverend Andrew Foster, an Afro-American, who had become totally deaf following meningitis at the age of 11, came to Ghana and obtained permission to set up a school for the "rehabilitation of the deaf and dumb" in Accra. The Reverend Foster conversed fluently by means of sign language and all his pupils were taught sign language. After an initial enrolment with 13 deaf children and 11 deaf adults, expansion was such that it was necessary to move the school to Mampong-Akwapim, about 30 km distant from Accra. There are two other schools for hearing-impaired children in Ghana. The Osu School for the Deaf in Accra is sponsored by the Ghana Society for the Deaf. It is a day school with 70 pupils who, because the teachers themselves have auditory impairments, are taught by the manual method. Younger pupils have full classroom instruction while a small amount of training is given to the older ones in basketry, carpentry, tailoring and sewing. The other school is at Wa in north-west Ghana. Here, the oral method of education is used. In 1965, a Deaf Education Specialist Training College was established at Mampong in association with the school there. The curriculum there is similar to that of the Department of Audiology and Education of the Deaf at the University of Manchester, but it has been modified to suit local needs so that all students learn dactylogy (Hewitt, 1968).

In Nigeria, the Society for the Care of the Deaf, which was founded in Lagos in January 1956, established the Federal School for the Deaf in 1957. By the time the civil war broke out (July, 1967) there were about half a dozen schools in Nigeria for the auditory handicapped, including schools in Ibadan and in Enugu. However, the educational systems suffered in that sign language was used or the pupils were taught to read and write in English only. However, at the Rehabilitation Centre and School for the Deaf which was set up at Enugu in 1961, a British teacher herself learned the Ibo language and taught children by oralism in their own language.

The Society for the Deaf in Sierra Leone was founded in 1962 (Luke and Renner-Lisk, 1968). The objects of the Society are "to promote the general welfare of the deaf and dumb in Sierra Leone through education, training and employment and to supply hearing aids in suitable cases". A school for the auditory handicapped was started by the Society in 1965 and now has 14 pupils. The Commonwealth Society for the Deaf has provided equipment for the school.

Fortunately, the normally hearing people in West Africa maintain a sympathetic attitude to those with auditory problems, and the younger people tend to look after the older people. Consequently, the auditory handicapped may not face such problems as they do in Europe and North America.

CONCLUSIONS

This survey has inevitably concentrated on Nigeria, but, with a population which exceeds that of all other West African states put together and encompassing diverse geographical areas, this country's neuro-otolaryngological problems reflect those of the rest of West Africa.

The pattern of neuro-otolaryngology is appreciably different from that of Europe or of North America. Nutritional factors have been proven in the aetiology or pathogenesis of a number of disorders, where auditory or vestibular disturbances may be only one facet of the general symptomatology. There are also good grounds for suspecting viruses as being aetiological factors, and some of these may have very lethal characteristics. Unfortunately, the size of the problems have yet to be ascertained. It would seem that future studies should first concentrate on surveys to determine the prevalence of the various disorders and epidemiological studies to ascertain the factors involved in the development of these disorders.

REFERENCES

Article (1970). *Daily Telegraph*, Feb. 11, p. 17.
Behrman, S. (1962). *Br. J. Ophthal.*, **46**, 554.
Borgstrom, G. A. (1969). "Too Many". Collier-Macmillan, London.
Brown, G. M. (1960). *Physiol. Rev.*, **40**, 331.
Buckley, S. M. and Casals, J. (1970). *Am. J. trop. Med. Hyg.*, **19**, 680.
Caddell, J. L. (1966). *Lancet*, **2**, 752.
Church, R. J. H. (1967). "Environment and Policies in West Africa". Van Nostrand. Princeton, N.J., U.S.A.
Collomb, H., Quere, M. A., Cros, J. and Giordano, C. (1967). *J. neurol. Sci.*, **5**, 159.
Collomb, H., Virieu, R., Dumas, M. and Tap, D. (1968). *Bull. Soc. Med. Afr. Langue Franc.*, **13**, 249.
Dada, T. O., Johnson, F. A., Araba, A. B. and Adegbite, S. A. (1969). *West Afr. Med. J.*, **18**, 95.

David, J. B., Edoo, B. B., Hinchcliffe, R. and Mustaffah, J. F. O. (1971). *Sound.* **5**, 70

Dumas, M., Tap, D., Vieillard, J. J. and Ayats, H. (1968). *Bull. Soc. Med. Afr. Langue Franc.*, **13**, 257.

Edoo, B. B. (1970). *Proc. II Pan-Afr. Congr. Neurol. Sci., Ibadan.*

Ekpechi, O. L. (1967). *Br. J. Nutr.*, **21**, 537.

Fiaxe, S. A. K. (1968). *In* "Commonwealth Society for the Deaf Report on the First Seminar on Deafness to be held in Africa", p. 86. Commonwealth Society for the Deaf, London.

Findlay, G. M. (1946). *Trans. R. Soc. trop. Med.*, **40**, 219.

Frame, J. D., Baldwin, J. M. Jr., Gocke, D. J. and Troup, J. M. (1970). *Am. J. trop. Med. Hyg.*, **19**, 670.

Girard, P. L., Courson, B. and Dumas, M. (1970). *Proc. II Pan-Afr. Congr. Neurol. Sci., Ibadan.*

Greenberg, J. H. (1963). *Internat. J. Am. Linguistics*, **29**, 1. Pt. II.

Hewitt, A. (1968). *In* "Commonwealth Society for the Deaf Report on the First Seminar on Deafness to be held in Africa", p. 83. Commonwealth Society for the Deaf, London.

Hill, K. R. (1952). *W. Ind. med. J.*, **1**, 243.

Hinchcliffe, R., Osuntokum, B. O. and Adeuja, A. O. G. (1971). *Audiology.* **11**, 2, 8

Ladefoged, P. (1968). "A Phonetic Study of West African Languages". Cambridge University Press, Cambridge.

Lagundoye, S. B. (1971). *Afr. J. Med. Sci.*, **2**, 121.

Luke, R. and Renner-Lisk, E. (1968). *In* "Commonwealth Society for the Deaf Report on the First Seminar on Deafness to be held in Africa", p. 94. Commonwealth Society for the Deaf, London.

Monekosso, G. L. and Wilson, J. (1966). *Lancet*, **1**, 1062.

Money, G. L. (1958). *W. Afr. Med. J.*, **7**, 58.

Nwokolo, C. and Ekpechi, O. L. (1966). *Trans. R. Soc. trop. Med. Hyg.*, **60**, 97.

Odeku, E. L. and Richard, D. R. (1970). *Proc. II Pan-Afr. Congr. Neurol. Sci., Ibadan.*

Odeku, E. L., Osuntokun, B. O., Adeloye, A. and Williams, A. O. (1970). *Proc. II Pan-Afr. Congr. Neurol. Sci., Ibadan.*

Oke, O. L. (1966). *Nature*, **212**, 1055.

Ormerod, F. (1961). "Survey of Deafness in Africa". Preliminary Report on a visit to East and West Africa. Unpublished Report to Colonial Office and Nuffield Trust.

Osuntokun, B. O. (1968). *Brain*, **91**, 215.

Osuntokun, B. O. (1969). Chronic cyanide intoxication and a Degenerative Neuropathy in Nigeria. Unpublished Ph.D. thesis. Univ. Ibadan, Nigeria.

Osuntokun, B. O. and Adeuja, A. O. G. (1970). *Proc. II Pan-Afr. Congr. Neurol. Sci., Ibadan.*

Osuntokun, B. O. and Williams, A. O. (1970). *Proc. II. Pan-Afr. Congr. Neurol. Sci., Ibadan.*

Osuntokun, B. O., Monekosso, G. L. and Wilson, J. (1969). *Br. Med. J.*, **1**, 547.

Osuntokun, B. O., Aladetoyinbo, A. and Adeuja, A. O. G. (1970). *Lancet*, **2**, 372.

Paula, G. de and Rangel, A. (1946). *Chem. Abr.*, **39**, 2161.

Pitres, A. (1895). *Rev. Med.*, **15**, 873.

Reynaud, J., Camara, M. and Basteris, L. (1969). *Int. Audiol.*, **8**, 299.

Simonetta, B. (1968). *Minerva Med.*, **59**, 4507.

Sinclair, H. M. and Jeliffe, D. B. (1961). *In* "Nicholls' Tropical Nutrition and Dieletics", p. 374. Baillière, Tindall and Cox, London.

Speir, R. W., Wood, O., Liebhaber, H. and Buckley, S. M. (1970). *Am. J. trop. Med. Hyg.*, **19**, 692.

Troup, J. M., White, H. A., Fom, A. L. M. D. and Carey, D. E. (1970). *Am. J. trop. Med. Hyg.*, **19**, 695.

Williams, A. O., Resch, J. A. and Loewenson, R. B. (1969). *Neurology*, **19**, 205.

Wright, J. and Morley, D. C. (1958). *Lancet*, **1**, 871.

Zigas, V. and Gajdusek, D. C. (1957). *Med. J. Australia*, **2**, 745.

Review of British Audiology

J. D. HOOD*

*Medical Research Council Hearing and Balance Unit,
Institute of Neurology, The National Hospital, London, England*

In reviewing British audiology, the terms of reference that have been given me are not to attempt some kind of personal assessment of selected topics of research being undertaken in Britain today. It would be imprudent of me to do so and in any event the participants of this Congress exemplify, in a way which could not be bettered, a fairly representative cross section of the individuals prominent in the field of audiology in Britain today and of the respective contributions they have made or are making. My task as I see it is rather to review British audiology in its much wider sense, to consider tour failings alongside our achievements and to attempt as best I can an outline of our future needs and requirements.

Although the term "audiology" was I believe first coined in 1939 by Hargrave, it would of course be quite wrong to suppose that before that time nothing was happening in this particular discipline in this or any other country. It is true that otologists were still largely pre-occupied with tuning-fork tests and clinical audiology as such was very much in its infancy, nevertheless the science of hearing was by no means a neglected subject. The physiology of hearing and the pathology and relief of deafness had formed important parts of the Medical Research Council's research programme for many years before the war and an advisory committee to direct work in this field had been appointed as long ago as 1928. This same committee later sponsored the issue of five reports dealing with such topics as the localization of sound, the use of hearing aids of the type then available in 1936 and with speech and hearing in children. These particular topics are of course as pertinent to us now as they were then.

I must confess I am not myself particularly familiar with the advances made at that time but the fact that these subjects were given considera-

* Past Chairman of the British Society of Audiology.

tion at all is a cautionary thought for those who might feel that by inventing a new discipline like audiology they have pioneered the way for an entirely new field of study. Prominent names that come to mind are those of Lord Adrian who made significant contributions to our knowledge of the cochlear microphonics, Dr T. S. Littler and Rawden Smith for their studies in auditory fatigue, Mr A. Tumarkin, and of course Dr C. S. Hallpike recently elected to honorary membership of the Society whose first papers in the field of audiology appeared early in the 1930s and have continued ever since.

No historical survey however would be complete without a special tribute to the Ewings' work at Manchester. To them goes the very special credit for having built the very solid foundations upon which the whole structure of paedo-audiology now rests. Sir Alexander Ewing is another of the honorary members of the Society and we are obliged to him for giving us such a distinguished first Thomas Simm Littler lecture. Under his guidance the Department of Audiology and Education of the Deaf grew from strength to strength and was I suppose the very first centre in this country devoted to organized research in audiology. The department is now under the very capable hands of Professor Ian Taylor and I am sure that Sir Alexander must take particular pride in the large and thriving establishment which now exists and which grew from such small beginnings.

The next landmark in audiology occurred in 1943 when towards the end of the war the Ministry of Health having in mind plans for a comprehensive National Health Service approached the Medical Research Council for help in dealing with the problems of deafness. As a result the Council took immediate action and formed their first unit on deafness, the Otological Research Unit under the direction of Dr C. S. Hallpike. This was followed in 1944 by the formation of three committees to deal with the various aspects of the prevention, treatment and relief of deafness. One of these committees, the so-called Electro-Acoustics Committee, was given the task amongst other things of determining the practicability of designing a single type of electrically operated hearing aid which would be small, and light to carry, reasonably cheap to produce and service, and capable of giving good intelligibility of the spoken word to the majority of persons with deafness of types that can be benefited by mechanical appliances. It is only right that I should mention that such a programme of work would probably not have been envisaged had it not been for the early pioneer work of the hearing-aid manufacturers in this country who can justly claim to be among the first in the field; in particular, the work of Edwin Stevens of Amplivox and the late Joseph Poliakoff of Multitone. The aims of the Electro-Acoustics Committee were directed at determining for the very first time the optimum frequency characteristic that a hearing aid should have.

To this end, two speech transmission systems were developed at the Post Office Research Station at Dollis Hill which enabled recorded lists of words or sentences to be delivered through telephones at a variety of sound pressure levels and with unlimited facilities for altering the frequency characteristics. One of these was installed at Manchester and the other at the National Hospital, Queen Square, where a deafness clinic came into being in association with the Otological Research Unit. At these two centres a crash programme of research was begun. I myself joined the unit at this time and can testify to the prodigious amount of effort by all concerned that went into this work.

The aim was to test as many patients as possible in the shortest possible time. Each patient was given a full otological examination and tested in a variety of ways with full speech audiometry and the best of the commercial hearing aids then available. The speech transmission system itself was equipped with four output channels so that four patients could be tested simultaneously. Difficult as it was the work was not without its lighter moments. The four patients being tested sat in a single room screened from each other by blanket-like material. In front of each sat a scorer whose task was to record the responses of the patients to each word delivered by the headphones. Unfortunately some of the patients had rather loud voices which could be heard from one cubicle to another so that not only had the scorers difficulty in determining the response of their particular charge but occasions arose when one patient repeating his version of the transmitted word, heard an adjoining patient's version of the same word and under the mistaken impression that he was being corrected by the scorer took it as something of a slight. The result was the somewhat hilarious situation of a kind of disembodied argument developing between two patients in adjoining cubicles under the impression that their adversaries were their respective scorers. In these circumstances the test had to be abandoned.

However, the result of all this was that an enormous amount of information was collected in a very short space of time and within a period of something like 18 months from the beginning of the programme the report was completed and presented to the Council. Its title was of course "Hearing Aids and Audiometers". The report is a classic of its type which has stood the test of time because the findings and conclusions it came to are as relevant now as they were then.

The report was followed in due course by the development and free issue of the Medresco Hearing Aid. So well had the Electro-Acoustics Committee done its job that the performance of this aid remains to this day second to none. In fact in the intervening years apart from miniaturization, advances in hearing aid design have been disappointingly small. The Electro-Acoustics Committee appreciated the fact that there would be a proportion of deaf people who would not derive benefit from the aid. They were not of course at that time in possession of the documented evidence we now have available to us of the disturbing effects of loudness recruitment in cochlear deafness. If they had I think it is extremely likely that something would have been done about it. As it is the electronic correction of deafness resulting from lesions of the cochlea remains one of our most pressing problems for which we have as yet no satisfactory solution.

The first years of the M.R.C. Otological Research Unit were taken up largely with the work of the Electro-Acoustics Committee but following upon the completion of the report Dr Hallpike embarked upon a programme of research concerned both with cochlear and vestibular function which continued until his retirement in 1965 and was responsible in no small measure, for laying the foundation of the speciality which has come to be known as neuro-otology. The advances in the audiological field were significant and far reaching and form the basis for many of the audiological test procedures now in current use.

Some years after the formation of the Otological Research Unit in 1949 the Medical Research Council formed a second research unit entitled the Werhner Research Unit on Deafness under the late Dr Littler, a man whose name the Society now commemorates in a Prize and a Lecture. Dr Littler had originally worked at the Department of Education of the Deaf at Manchester with Sir Alexander Ewing and was the secretary of the Electro-Acoustics Committee, a post he held for many years after the publication of the report, until in fact the committee was disbanded. The unit was originally housed at the Royal National Throat Nose and Ear Hospital at Golden Square and later moved to Kings College Hospital at Denmark Hill where it remained until its disbandonment on Dr Littler's retirement in 1965. This unit was the training ground for a number of people whose names are now household words in British audiology.

The late Edith Whetnall who made such distinguished contributions in paedo-audiology and was largely responsible for the formation of the Nuffield Hearing and Speech Centre at Gray's Inn Road was for a time associated with the unit. Our present chairman, vice-chairman and treasurer, Dr Hinchcliffe, Dr Knight and Dr Coles, were members of the staff together with Dr Ralph Naunton who is now Professor of Otology at Chicago University. It is perhaps not surprising that the Society holds Dr Littler's name in such high esteem.

I shall have more to say of the work of the Werhner Research Unit presently but I have dealt with it here at some length together with Manchester and the Otological Research Unit because for a considerable period of time after the war these were the only centres where any organized form of audiological work was being carried out and to this extent all three have played an influential role in moulding audiology in Britain as it is today.

Nowadays, matters are very different and from those small beginnings, interest in audiology has grown at an astonishing rate, particularly within the last ten years. I mentioned earlier that work in a particular field does not necessarily have its origin at that moment in time when the field of study is given a label like "Audiology". Nevertheless, there can be no doubt that once a particular discipline has received recognition, the respectability thereby imparted to it does much to encourage activity in that field and this has surely been the case with audiology.

This brings me to the subject of the British Society of Audiology. The Society was founded largely upon the initiative of our present chairman, Dr R. Hinchcliffe, who early in 1967 gathered together a small number of individuals prominent in audiology who were later to form the provisional Council of the Society. The Inaugural Meeting was held in September 1967 and at that time with much perseverance we had been able to muster an initial membership of about 90. There were some who had doubts about the need for a society devoted solely to audiology and took the view that our needs could be met by sharing the activities of kindred societies. However the fact that in less than four years our membership has grown to 470* and continues to grow month by month is clear enough evidence of the need for a British Society of Audiology.

Today I think we can look back upon the first four years of the Society's history with some satisfaction. To a very large extent we have achieved our principle aim namely to provide a forum for the exchange of ideas in all branches of audiology. Our regular meetings and symposia have been well attended and ranged over a wide field. In addition the Scottish and Northern branches of the Society formed more recently have been particularly successful due in no small measure to the active and vigorous leadership of their respective chairmen and secretaries.

The formation of the Society has served to reveal to us for the first time the wealth of audiological research being carried out in this country. Before it existed I was unaware of the considerable activity being carried out in this field. *Sound*, The British Journal of Audiology

---

* Present membership is 518.

which was the brain child of Air Vice-Marshal Dickson, Chairman of the R.N.I.D., the third of our honorary members, is now the official organ of the Society in which are published the Society proceedings. The high standard which this journal has been able to maintain over the past few years is itself a tribute to the Society and the workers in the field of audiology.

When one considers the paucity of financial support given to audiological research only ten years ago I would hazard a guess that in recent years it has increased by at least a factor of ten. In this connection I feel confident that the formation of the Society has played some part in drawing attention to the need for research in hearing and deafness. There remains of course much to be desired. We have as yet no single centre that can match in size or resources any one of a number of such centres that are to be found in the States. I don't know whether or not the authorities have some feelings of guilt about this but in the Chronically Sick and Disabled Persons Bill that was passed through Parliament last year Clause 24 reads as follows:

> The Secretary of State shall collate and present evidence to the Medical Research Council on the need for an institute for hearing research, such institute to have the general function of co-ordinating and promoting research on hearing and assistance to the deaf and hard of hearing.

Many of us have already been interviewed on this topic so that it would seem that some action is being taken. There are, however, as is to be expected, a number of conflicting views. In a symposium which Mr Jack Ashley, M.P., persuaded the CIBA Foundation to hold on the subject of Sensori-neural Hearing Loss in 1969 Dr Fisch offered the following comments:

> According to a certain school of thought, new ideas leading to a real breakthrough usually occur accidentally and therefore a concerted and planned effort is a waste of time. I entirely disagree with this view. It is true that many new discoveries have been made seemingly accidentally, but often it was not as accidental as it seemed. These discoveries occur in a certain atmosphere of thought and in a certain environment which made such an accident possible; usually it was not accidental that this atmosphere or environment was created. The probability of such a discovery being made was very high. On the other hand, many discoveries have been made as a result of a deliberately planned and concerted effort.
>
> We have come to a cross-roads in our search for better understanding of some of the fundamental problems of sensori-neural deafness. We have made great advances by research in little bits and pieces, carried out by individuals or small isolated groups. Although these efforts will always be valuable, it seems to me that unless the best resources of science are made available to multidisciplinary research teams it is unlikely that we shall

make a significant advance within a reasonable time. We cannot afford to wait passively for accidental discoveries to drop suddenly into our laps. Those who are engaged in this work feel this very strongly and are very disappointed by the lack of support and understanding in this respect. The reasons for this go much deeper than are generally appreciated. There is such a thing in the society as a hierarchy of human disabilities. Some disabilities, for various reasons, are considered more important and deserving more sympathy and more material support than others. A recent investigation was made to test public opinion on which disability was considered more, or less, important and deserving more, or less, support. Deafness was almost at the bottom of the list. There are then deeper social reasons why deafness, which is one of the major disabilities, is not supported to a greater extent.

By contrast Dr Nelson Kiang at the same symposium after making the point that it was important to enlist the aid of what he called first class brains in this country went on to say:

It is not that I am against a special institute; I do not know enough about it. What I am saying is that an institute would be irrelevant. It does not matter whether you have an institute or not, the important factor is to get good brains into the field. If an institute is to be set up, the most important thing is to remove from it, as much as possible, the influence of medical politics. The trouble with so many organizations that are started from the top down is that they become immediately involved in politics. I am not saying that this will necessarily happen, but one must minimize the influence of politics in research and allow scientific truth to be the criterion of success. There is really no difference between clinical research and basic research. They both come down to the question of when do you know something, and the same rules of inquiry hold for both endeavours.

Be this as it may there is one important problem that faces us which has some relevance to it. In my inaugural address to the Society in 1967 I said:

There is much profit to be had from the active integration of the results of studies in these two fields of audiology, the clinical and the non-clinical. All too frequently the clinical audiologist is unappreciative of the advances made by the physiologist, the psychologist, the physicist and others, while conversely those working in the non-clinical field are often unaware of the problems posed in clinical audiology.

One of our functions will be to encourage active co-operation and exchange of ideas in these two branches of audiology. If we meet with only partial success in this respect our efforts in founding this Society will have been well rewarded.

In this respect I do not think the Society can as yet claim to have made much headway and these two aspects of audiological research seem to be as far removed as ever. Electro-physiologists, for example, in this and other contries are carrying out outstanding fundamental research on hearing mechanisms, nevertheless I can think of no single outcome of their investigations that has directly resulted in any way in the alleviation of deafness. The phenomenon of loudness recruitment is a case in point. We now know a very great deal about its psycho-physical aspects but very little about its patho-physiology and yet such a knowledge could be of enormous help to us both in its treatment and also in hearing-aid design.

It might or might not be that an Institute of Hearing Research by bringing together all the various disciplines could be the stimulus for a single-minded attack on the many problems of deafness that still await a solution. It is, however, of no use saying we must attract the best brains in the country if all we can offer them are problems to be solved without providing them with the proper environment and the wherewithal for doing it.

While on the subject of hopes and aspirations let me return to something else I said in my inaugural address as follows:

> In the important field of clinical audiology there is much to be done. In the otological departments of the medical schools of this country, apart from a very few enlightened centres, audiology remains a much neglected subject, and few otologists in training are given the opportunity to make themselves conversant with modern audiological techniques.

This situation has improved somewhat since 1967 largely through the initiative of the younger otologists but not so rapidly as one would have wished. In part, the problem stems from the fact that there is a dearth of lecturers in audiology with the necessary clinical experience competent to teach at post-graduate level.

It is particularly welcome news therefore to hear that certain centres at Manchester, Salford and Southampton are organizing M.Sc. courses in audiology. These courses will in time fulfil a much felt need not only, one would hope, for the use the medical schools will be able to make of them, but also in providing personnel to take charge of the larger regional audiological establishments which one hopes will develop in the course of time within the National Health Service. Of course, viewed in the light of our existing audiological services all this may seem so much wishful thinking to many engaged in this kind of work.

Audiology in the past has never been high in the Department of Health's list of priorities and in particular a review of the salaries and conditions of service of the audiology technician is long overdue.

There are at the present time over 200 audiology technicians employed within the National Health Service. Like certain other dedicated professions they are a devoted and overworked branch of people prepared to sacrifice financial considerations in the interests of work for the community. However praiseworthy this may be it is not the best foundation upon which to build a sound audiological service. What is needed is first and foremost a substantial increase both in their salary and in their numbers. In addition it is absolutely essential that they should undertake a suitable course of instruction and be properly qualified. Many of them have, of course, attended audiology courses of the kind at present held at Gray's Inn Road and taken the examination prescribed by the Society of Audiology Technicians. Unfortunately, the possession of such a qualification at the present time carries with it little professional advantage because as a result of a circular issued by the Department of Health in 1965 the grading of audiology technicians is determined only by a certificate of competence issued by the otologist in charge without any requirement for the technicians to have attended an approved course.

This kind of situation is unsatisfactory both for the otologist and the technician firstly, because there exists no incentive for the technician to advance his knowledge in audiology and secondly, it is impossible to maintain a uniformly high standard of competence throughout the country let alone attempt to improve it. This is in rather ludicrous contrast to the Standard of Competence announced by the recently formed Hearing Aid Council for Hearing Aid Dispensers. The Hearing Aid Council you will recall is the outcome of the Hearing Aid Council Act which that indefatigable champion of the deaf, Mr Laurie Pavitt, pioneered through Parliament in 1968. The Council's standard of competence requires that in future all hearing-aid dispensers must, after undertaking an approved course of study pass an appropriate examination. I have seen the syllabus for this examination and it is remarkably similar to that of the Society of Audiology Technicians.

We have, therefore, the anomalous position of the commercial sector of audiology insisting upon a qualification by examination for its dispensers not required by the National Health Service for its technicians. Important as the dispensing of hearing aids may be it is surely subservient to the audiology service the otologist and the public at large have a right to expect from the N.H.S. How far the implementation of the Zuckerman report will alter the present position remains to be seen, but in any event I think it is encouraging to note that the Department of Health are aware of the need for action in this sphere.

I should like to turn now to an event of some importance to British audiology which took place last year, namely the publication by the Stationery Office of the report "Hearing and Noise in Industry" by Professor Burns and Dr D. W. Robinson. This report has an extraordinary long history which dates back to 1957 when, following upon discussions with the then Department of Scientific and Industrial Research, the late Dr T. S. Littler, in collaboration with the two authors, submitted a scheme of research aimed at a field study of occupational hearing loss with a view to evolving quantitative relations between noise exposure and deterioration of hearing.

It was not until 1961 that Treasury approval was finally given and in 1962 the Medical Research Council and the National Physical Laboratory were allocated the responsibility for carrying out the investigations.

The data were obtained over the five years 1963 to 1968 during which time some 4,000 hearing tests were carried out with the aid of a mobile laboratory especially equipped for the purpose.

Both our chairman and vice-chairman, Dr Hinchcliffe and Dr Knight, played a prominent part in obtaining this information which must surely have been a particularly arduous task for all concerned. The end result however is a unique and outstanding achievement which should have far reaching legislative and medical consequences. The essence of the report rests in the fact that to a given noise environment can now be ascribed, simply and rapidly, definite properties which, taken in conjunction with the duration of the exposure, enable specific degrees of hearing loss distributed in a particular way over the exposed population to be predicted.

In other words the assessment of risk to hearing can as a result of the information presented in the report be assessed in clear statistical terms; noisy occupations can be rated according to the degree of hearing risk to the workers and such remedial action as is necessary, instituted. It is not without significance that coincidental with the publication of the report the Industrial Injuries Advisory Council appointed a sub-committee to advise on the prescription of occupational hearing loss as an industrial injury. The Society together with many other bodies gave evidence to this committee which is now considering the matter. Whatever conclusions they come to there is no doubt that they have been set a very difficult task.

Not the least of the problems they will have to get to grips with are how one makes the diagnosis of occupational hearing loss, how deafness relates to social disability and how it is to be compensated. In addition one wonders how the already overstrained otological services will be able to cope with the flood of patients which is likely to result from the prescription of occupational hearing loss and for that matter how the staff will be found to carry out the essential audiological tests. These are difficult problems for which a solution will have to be found in due course.

I have tried as best I could to review the present state of British audiology as I see it. No doubt there are a number of omissions in what

1 have had to say, but the field is such a wide one involving so many disciplines, that I doubt if any review could be completely comprehensive and on this score I hope I will be forgiven if I have left unsaid any of the things I should have said. I cannot end, however, without paying a very special tribute to the President of the Conference, Dr Taylor. The Society owes him a very special vote of thanks for the tremendous amount of effort and hard work he devoted to making the Conference such a success. It was the first conference of the British Society of Audiology and set a standard both in its organization and execution which the Society will be hard pressed to maintain in the years to come.

As to the future I think we can look forward with considerable confidence. I mentioned earlier that one of the outcomes of the formation of the Society was the revelation of the considerable and, to some extent, unknown amount of work of high quality being carried out in this field.

Perhaps the most encouraging aspect of this is that much of this work is being undertaken by young enthusiasts *despite* the lack of direct financial support rather than as a result of it. I think this is extremely important because it clearly demonstrates, if such a demonstration were needed, that there exists both the enthusiasm and the ability to carry out audiological research in this country. What seems to be needed now is some authoritative action, backed by financial support, to harness it into a concerted attack upon the many problems of hearing and deafness that still await a solution.

Closing Remarks

RONALD HINCHCLIFFE

Institute of Laryngology and Otology, University of London, London, England

Over the past few days, the evidence has been presented that British Audiology has come to stay. For the opportunity to present this evidence we are grateful to our Conference President, Dr William Taylor, who with his colleagues, has ensured that this has been a happy and informative occasion.

For three days, Dundee has been a home for British and International Audiologists. We must now disperse. There are those of us, however, who hope for a permanent home for British Audiology, which could form a base for people with special training and experience who could continue to serve the auditory handicapped with devotion, diligence and dignity; a vision of our future where neither those who serve nor those who are served will merit the stigma of the underprivileged. The necessary enactment is now on the Statute Book of this country. May it be implemented.

Author Index

Numbers in *italics* are those pages where references are listed

263

Subject Index